Barbara Hannah

the CAT DOG *and* HORSE LECTURES

Barbara Hannah

the CAT DOG *and* HORSE LECTURES

"THE BEYOND"

IN TUNE WITH THE UNCONSCIOUS
A Portrait of Barbara Hannah

by

Dean L. Frantz and Ann Wintrode

Chiron Publications
Asheville, North Carolina

www.chironpublications.com

Library of Congress Catalog Card Number: 92-15830

Printed in the United States of America.
Book design by Siobhan Drummond.
Cover design by Michael Barron.

Library of Congress Cataloging-in-Publication Data:

Hannah, Barbara.
[Lectures. Selections]
Barbara Hannah : the cat, dog, and horse lectures, and "The beyond" / edited by Dean L. Frantz ; In tune with the unconscious : a portrait of Barbara Hannah by Dean L. Frantz and Ann Wintrode.
p. cm.
Includes bibliographical references and index.
ISBN 978-1-63051-514-0
1. Archetype (Psychology) 2. Cats—Psychological aspects. 3. Dogs—Psychological aspects. 4. Horses—Psychological aspects. 5. Future life—Psychological aspects. 6. Hannah, Barbara.
I. Wintrode, Ann. II. Frantz, Dean L. III. Title.
BF109.H345A5 1992
150.19'54—dc20 92-15830
CIP

ISBN 978-1-63051-514-0

CONTENTS

PREFACE

This book includes six of Barbara Hannah's unpublished lectures, along with an essay, "The Beyond." These writings will give the reader a glimpse of the depth and breadth of this woman who was associated with Jung for thirty years and who wrote the biography, *Jung, His Life and Work: A Biographical Memoir.* In her ninety-five years, she achieved a high degree of wholeness.

I first met Miss Hannah in 1968 and saw her for the last time in 1985. My reflections after her death make clear my deep respect for her, as well as the importance of my relationship with her for almost two decades. When she was ninety-two, I was prompted by my dreams and by suggestions from friends to get her consent to write about her life. Although somewhat reluctant to undertake such a task at her age, she finally agreed to work with me on this project.

The portrait presented here is all too brief because Barbara Hannah was secretive about her life and modest about her achievements. But I have tried to include the important chapters of her life and, above all, to portray her commitment to the unconscious, which is at the heart of Jung's psychology.

One of the fringe benefits of my years of working with Miss Hannah was a fund of statements from Jung, stories about him which throw light on his psychology, and some stories of her own, all of which, to my knowledge, have not been previously published. They are included here in the portrait of Barbara Hannah, as a means of shedding additional light on the life and thought of Barbara Hannah and Jung himself.

—Dean L. Frantz

Chronology of the Life of Barbara Hannah

August 2, 1891	Birth
1891–1902	Early childhood in Brighton, England
1902–1909	Adolescence in Chichester, England
1907	Death of her mother
1914–1918	Nursing duty in World War I
1918–1929	Travel and study
1929	Arrival in Zürich
January 14, 1929	First interview with C. G. Jung
1931	Death of her father
1934	Drawing of Jung's portrait
1952	First trip to America
June 6, 1967	Memorial lecture at the C. G. Jung Institute of Zürich
1968	Second trip to America for the Bailey Island Conference
1971	Publication of *Striving Toward Wholeness*
1976	Publication of *Jung, His Life and Work: A Biographical Memoir*
1981	Publication of *Encounters with the Soul: Active Imagination*
September 4, 1986	Death

IN TUNE WITH THE UNCONSCIOUS

A Portrait of Barbara Hannah

by Dean L. Frantz

THE FORMATIVE YEARS

If a mother can communicate prenatally with her child, as some research suggests, then Barbara Hannah may have been listening in the womb when her mother said, "The doctor tells me I'm going to have another baby, but I really don't want the little beast." Perhaps this rejection contributed to the fact that Barbara's weight at six months was exactly what it had been at birth. When Jung heard this story many years later, he commented, "Barbara must have wondered if she had come to the right place."

The place to which she came was Brighton, England, where her father was a pastor, as was his father before him. The Hannah family, long-time Methodists, had lived in Lincolnshire in southern Scotland for four hundred years. Barbara's grandfather was the first to leave Scotland, as well as the first to break away from the Methodist Church and join the Church of England.

The child born August 2, 1891, to Annie Barbara and John Julius Hannah, was given the name of Juliet Barbara, the middle names of her parents. For six years she was called by the Gaelic name of Sheila, but when a rare dog, also named Sheila, was given to the family, it was clear that "something had to give." The dog kept the name of Sheila, and Juliet Barbara became known as Barbara. Her first name was never used again.

The youngest of five children, Barbara had a sister and three brothers. Because of her mother's social responsibilities as the wife of a vicar, and later a dean, she was reared largely by nurses and governesses.

When Barbara was twelve, her mother found some of her poems and was so impressed that she wanted to have them published. Because her mother "made a fuss" over the poems, she stopped writing verse. "I'll paint," she said, and paint she did until she was thirty-seven. "I didn't know why but I had to express something I wasn't expressing in ordinary life," she said.

*Jung told about a man who had a strong mother complex. After his analytical hours, the man would write details to his mother, with whom he lived. Jung told him this had to stop or he would terminate the analysis. The man dreamed his mother went up a steep hill, slipped and broke her leg. The next day Jung got a telegram from the man saying that his mother had indeed broken her leg.**

When you are tempted to think critically, ask if it can be done another way. If not, then go ahead.

However, what Barbara's mother did, as a whole, must not have been all bad. Jung said that he had never known a case where a mother did so little harm to her children. Many mothers would settle for such a tribute. Her mother died of cancer in May 1907, when Barbara was fifteen. Barbara said that as she grew up, she liked her mother very much and was "enormously saddened" by her death.

About her father, Barbara said: "He was rather a nice man. I quite understand that. Women liked him very much but he was not a good father." However, she was grateful to him for keeping animals, especially horses. She said that she learned to ride before she learned to walk. When she was slow to begin walking (choosing rather to move on all fours) her father said, "If that child won't walk, I'll teach her to ride." She credited him with her life-long love of horses and other animals. As a child, she especially liked the spirited ponies. At age three, when she got on a pony that reared and the protecting groom removed her, she bit the

---

*Marginalia are quotes from Barbara Hannah.

groom! (She was confined to bed the rest of the day and never bit anyone else.)

Barbara's childhood was divided into the years before the age of eleven, when she lived in Brighton, and the years after eleven, when she lived in Chichester, where her father was Dean of Chichester Cathedral. She described her Brighton days as happy, even though she was lonely and sick much of the time, but she hated Chichester from the beginning.

She disliked being forced to go to church services when attendance was low and bodies were needed to fill the pews—sometimes three times a day. On occasion she would arrive during the last hymn, and the verger would seat her at the end of a pew toward the back of the church. After the service she would mingle with the crowd, and her father never knew she had not attended the entire service.

If a person has a religious experience and it is genuine for him, that is fine. But if he tries to enforce it upon others, that becomes inflation.

As a young man, Barbara's father had wanted to study law; when his mother threatened to cut him out of her will unless he went into the ministry, he followed her wishes, but without enthusiasm. Barbara said, "He wasn't ever fully in it." He was unhappy with his profession from the beginning, and late in life admitted that there was little conviction behind his words from the pulpit.

An incident involving her father when Barbara was a teenager brought her mixed messages from the adult world. One day, her father left the barn door open and his horse got out and wrecked Barbara's bicycle. When her father refused to repair the bicycle, Barbara became distressed. She confided in a friend of her mother who suggested that Barbara withhold a small amount from the grocery money each month until she accumulated enough to repair the bicycle. Barbara, somewhat aghast, asked, "But isn't that dishonest?" Her mother's friend replied, "It's not a question of honesty; we're talking about how to handle difficult men." When Barbara told this story to Jung, he said that that was a woman he would have liked to know, a woman who knew about Eros.

After the death of her mother, Barbara went with her father on a boat trip to Iceland and Norway. She said that on the trip she discovered what a tyrant he was. She especially resented his refusing to let her have her inheritance from her mother. She did not get the money until she was twenty-seven years old.

Barbara had only one term in high school because her mother thought the school ruined her English. At seventeen, two years after her mother's death, she entered a finishing school for four terms. She then studied art for a time at the Westminster School of Art in London with her long-time friend Constance Bailward.

At the outbreak of World War I, Barbara chose to serve as a nurse in the hospital at Chichester. Although she had no formal training as a nurse, she received enough instruction to enable her to be useful in that time of emergency. She was assigned to the children's ward where she was responsible for seventy-two beds. She described the work as difficult but said that she hated it most when they were not busy. During the war years, she took time off to be with her father when he went to Philpott, their country home.

BROADENING HORIZONS

After the war, Barbara studied art for a time at the Westminster School of Art in London with Constance Bailward. Constance was a sister of John Bailward, to whom Barbara was "more or less engaged for several years." As children, Constance and Barbara had shared a governess, the girls living half a year with the Bailward family and half a year with the Hannahs. Their friendship began when they were twelve and continued until they were about thirty. Constance was a wealthy young woman who shared Barbara's interest in art and who sponsored Barbara on their travels to paint and study. Barbara was reluctant to accept such generosity, but Constance convinced Barbara that she (Constance) could not go alone. Also, the traveling gave Barbara an opportunity to establish her freedom from her father and to pursue her artistic goals.

Their artistic adventures began in London and took them to Paris, Rome, Tunis, and back to Paris. Then Constance married and Barbara was left alone in Paris. One day she decided that there were enough paintings in the world and that she would not continue to increase the number. She gave up painting as her principal activity as suddenly as she started it.

PRELUDE TO ZÜRICH

In *Encounters with the Soul* Barbara wrote, "Jung saw that very little, if anything, happens 'by chance.' "[1] So it was not by chance that someone gave Barbara Hannah (who knew nothing of Carl Jung) a copy of his *Psychological Types*, which she read with great interest. A year later she discovered an article by Jung entitled "Woman in Europe." She read half the article and realized that if she finished it, it might change her life. Not sure that she was ready to change, she put the article away and went to her studio. Unable to concentrate on her painting, she went back at lunchtime and finished the article.

Jung said the difference between Indian women and European women was that the former dressed beautifully, but the latter reminded him of a wet hen before breakfast.

Jung spoke of the basic difference between men and women. He said if a match box floated in the air and forgot the law of gravity, men would say it didn't really happen, but women would crowd around to see this irrational event.

"It just made me feel that life was on a different basis from what I thought," she said. "This man knows something that nobody else knows. There IS something in life after all." Immediately she ordered all of Jung's books that were published in English.

---

[1]Barbara Hannah, *Encounters with the Soul: Active Imagination* (Santa Monica, Calif.: Sigo Press, 1981), p. 10.

Jung spoke of God's kindness in sending the gift of a neurosis, which often turns out to be a blessing in disguise.

Jung's books caused Barbara to recognize that there was something wrong with her life. Her doctor referred her to a Freudian psychiatrist, but there was no rapport. She left before the hour was over because of what she termed "senseless conversation." "Now I go to Jung," she said.

But the book that really sent Barbara to Jung was *Two Essays* which gives an overview of analytical psychology and attempts to establish the "independence of the unconscious." The unconscious was to become the guiding principle of her life.

The unconscious wants to say something to us—it may also want to ask us questions.

Two significant encounters with the unconscious occurred when Barbara was living alone in Paris. A brother of John Bailward, Barbara's fiancé, told Barbara that John had fallen in a hunting accident and broken his leg. Barbara thought, "My God, now I suppose I must go back and look after him." That night, the unconscious spoke to Barbara in the form of a vision of a tall archetypal woman who asked, "What is the most important thing in your life?" To Barbara's amazement, she heard herself say, "To help humanity around the corner that confronts it." Then the woman said, "If that's what you want, then leave John."

In recalling this vision years later, Barbara said:

> I didn't know anything about such things in those days, but it was something I felt to be an order. I knew I had to obey this woman. I didn't know anything about the Self; I only knew I had to take this woman seriously. I knew nothing about psychology at the time; now I know the woman was an archetype of the Self. I never went back to England to John.

The way of certainty is not the way of life.

Breaking with John was a major decision for Barbara because their marriage plans had been firm enough that they had discussed the seriousness of bringing children into an uncertain world. Even so, she now knew that she had to accept the message from the unconscious.

The unconscious is like nature: kind and terrible, loving and revengeful.

Then she had a dream about passing through British customs on her way to Switzerland. She was terrified that she would not be allowed to leave the country, but a woman appeared who told the customs officials that Barbara was traveling with her. In the dream, Barbara realized that she would accompany this woman on her journey, and there would be no turning back (this dream is reported on p. 291 in *Striving Toward Wholeness,* but the dreamer is not identified).

This same woman appeared in another dream and told Barbara to "go down to Zürich." Later she had the following dream, which confirmed her decision to go to Zürich.

> *I was in a big steamer and that steamer was Paris. I was not at all happy there. A small boat appeared, and I knew that I must jump into the small boat. The sea was rough. I thought, "Those are the Zürich people. I'll jump and they will catch me." I jumped but the people disappeared. However, I landed safely on my feet and said, "This is the way for me."*

Shortly after this dream, she wrote to Jung and asked for an appointment. Although she received no answer, she was not to be deterred. She wrote again, telling Jung that she was coming to Zürich and requesting that he refer her to someone if he could not see her. Fortunately, she left for Zürich without waiting for his answer, which turned out to be discouraging. As she stood on the train platform waiting for the night train to Zürich, she felt that she was on the verge of a drastic change in her life. On the train, she dreamed of an iron door closing behind her, and she knew that she would not be able to open it.

THE JOURNEY BEGINS

Barbara's first interview with Jung, described in detail in her biography of him, took place on January 14, 1929. While she was waiting to see Jung, she had a hypnagogic vision of four priests in a wood forming a square. She sketched a mandala of this vision.

At first, Jung tried to discourage Barbara from coming to Zürich. He praised her talent for drawing and urged her to return to Paris and continue her art. But when she told him of her dreams prior to coming to Zürich, he said: "It is really serious, isn't it? I see you have to put in your lot with us." (Later, when Barbara asked Jung why he had not answered her first letter, he said: "I saw from your letter that if you came to Zürich, it would change your whole life. I wasn't going to give you any help on that; you had to do it yourself.")

Jung seldom took beginners as analysands. After seeing Barbara twice, he turned her over to Toni Wolff, who later referred her to Peter Baynes. She analyzed with Toni and Peter for about two years and also worked with Emma Jung one summer. Barbara had this to say about Toni Wolff:

> She was an exceptional woman, so unlike anyone else. It was not by chance that Jung met her. She succeeded in finding the Self but left out the shadow. Jung helped her discover her shadow for his own sake as well as for hers. While Jung was doing his exploration of the unconscious, he often got into difficult areas, and Toni was able to keep him calm. Toni once said that Jung had so come to terms with his anima that you could appeal to him on his masculine or feminine side—that he was the only person she ever knew who was both a man and a woman.

The only things that stick with people are the things they get themselves.

At sixty years of age, Jung said, "Growing up is giving up childishness." At eighty, he still felt that way. An incident involving Emma Jung illustrated how Jung reacted to his wife's childishness. During World War II, Barbara Hannah arranged to get a special permit for extra gasoline rations so she could drive Jung to lectures rather than have him expend the effort required to take the train. But Emma Jung, thinking it would cause all kinds of gossip, "raised a fuss" and cancelled Barbara's arrangements. When Jung asked Emma why she had done this, she explained, then relented of her rashness, and said that it was all right for Barbara to drive Jung. But Jung put his foot down and said, "No, I am not going to let you change it now." Whenever he took the train into Zürich, he insisted that his wife watch him, in order to raise the level of her consciousness.

If one goes into the Grand Canyon, one should take all necessary precautions.

ANALYSIS WITH JUNG

Perhaps one of the greatest things that the unconscious did for Barbara was to get her into analysis with Jung. Help came in the form of a dream:

> *I was riding a horse and fell into a deep ditch. Toni seized one of my legs and Peter the other. I realized there was no way of escaping unless I could make Jung hear my cries for help. Jung was working in a field several fields away. I yelled at the top of my voice, hoping he would hear.*

Peter Baynes had the good sense to send Barbara to Jung with this dream. When Jung heard the dream, he said, "They couldn't manage it, I didn't think they could."

Barbara's analysis and close association with Jung, which began in 1931, spanned a period of thirty years. Initially, she saw Jung twice a week, then once a week, and finally only when she had a dream that she did not understand.

Our own dreams are difficult to understand because we dream in our own shadow.

"When I first saw Jung," Barbara said, "I saw the first person I'd ever seen whom I could trust entirely, and I thought, whatever he says, I'll do. I had never felt that way about anybody."

Jung once said to her, "You trust me more than anybody does."

"More than Toni?" she asked.

"Oh, much more than Toni," Jung replied. He said that it almost alarmed him that she trusted him so much.

Near the beginning of her analysis, Barbara dreamed of a beautiful rainbow. Jung told her that it represented the union of opposites, a symbol of what was at the end of the road, but that in between she could expect to travel through dirt and mud and muck. One of her dreams that emphasized the opposites is reported in *Striving Toward Wholeness* (p. 297), but the dreamer is not identified.

Jung said his job was to help people live the middle way between the opposites.

The road to individuation has many detours and turnings.

The individuation process always leads to an insoluble problem.

You may not do certain things yourself, but you have a way of attracting them, and the net effect is the same.

Individuation calls for a strong moral standpoint but not necessarily straitlaced!

Jung did not advocate shock therapy or hypnosis. He said, "Let the unconscious provide its own shock."

In a seminar, Jung said, "You think you have the worst problem in the world and nobody could have a worse one. You are right; yours is the most difficult because it is yours."

The individuation process does not have a sensible goal; it is like walking in the dark.

A jealous wife can stand prostitutes, and the cheapest kind of companions, anything but another decent woman.

When she asked Jung why he had taken her as an analysand, he said, "I knew you were a good cup and would not break easily." But like all analysands who take their analysis seriously, there were times when she thought she would "break." Jung used to tell her that when she thought she was through the worst of it, the worst was probably still ahead.

Once she dreamed of a burglar. When she told this dream to Jung, he said: "I always thought you were above that, but now I know you are capable of it. However, as your consciousness has darkened, it has also widened, and that is the important thing."

At one time, when she was struggling with a bad conscience, Jung said to her, "There will come a time when you will say, 'Damned if I care if I'm wrong' and then it will be all right." On another occasion she told Jung, "I've always heard 'Do this' or 'Do that.' " He answered, "After awhile you will get tired of it, and then you will say, 'To hell with it.' "

During the course of her analysis, she learned the basic psychological truth that everything beautiful also has its dark side. Once she had a lovely dream, but the next day she confessed a terrible thing. She said that some of the best things Jung did for her were "nasty" at the time, but that later they proved to be helpful.

When interviewed for biographical material, Barbara said, "I'm not going to tell you anything about my analysis or my individuation process; that's between Jung and me." However, she did mention two areas of difficulty that help us identify with her as a human being in spite of her extraordinary achievement in individuation.

Barbara once told Jung that she couldn't help being jealous of Ruth Bailey, Jung's housekeeper and long-time family friend, and of Dr. von Franz, who helped Jung so much with his alchemy research. Jung answered her by asking, "What do YOU do?" She said, "I give lectures and I have more people who want to analyze with me than I can take, but these are not things I do with you." Jung explained that what she was doing was just as important to him as cooking his food or whatever.

Another undesirable trait that Barbara claimed to have, which might be questioned by those who knew her, was laziness. At ninety-three, she said, "My chief thing is laziness." She said she "felt awful" when Jung told her from time to time: "You would be entirely individuated if you had taken enough time, but as it is, you always get a bit lazy at it." She remarked that most people in their mid-nineties probably feel that they have done enough and need not do any more. "I don't feel that way, so I have to fight my laziness. I've got a very lazy streak," she insisted.

There could be no Sahara without grains of sand. There could be no ocean without drops of water.

Only the person approaching individuation knows how intolerable man is to himself.

Jung asked a girl with whom he was working in analysis, "Don't you have a boyfriend?" She replied, "Yes, but I am committed to analysis." Jung responded, "You do not have a commitment to analysis. You have a commitment to life. Get married and come back later."

DEATH OF HER FATHER

Barbara was in analysis with Jung when word came that her father was seriously ill. Although she had "fought passionately" with her father for twenty years, she had made peace with him a year or so before his final illness.

She considered going to her father before he died. Then she dreamed that a huge oak tree in the forest fell and crushed a young beech tree growing nearby. When she told Jung the dream, he said, "I will not tell you not to go see your father before he dies, but it is very risky." She returned to England after her father's death.

The first night after the funeral she dreamed that she ate her father's shoulder. When she told this puzzling dream to Jung, he was horrified at first. Then he commented: "His death could eat you. It is better that you eat him first." Barbara was thirty-nine when her father died.

RELATIONSHIP WITH JUNG

Barbara developed a special and enviable relationship with Jung apart from her association with him as an analysand. She was fortunate to be invited to Bollingen three times the first year she was in Zürich. Over the years, she became a frequent visitor to Bollingen, which she described as "a place beyond all others."

Barbara went to Bollingen often to sketch for the pencil drawing of Jung that she drew for his sixtieth birthday. She did the portrait at Jung's request. Because she drew him while he was "occupied with his own work," the portrait presented him "in a totally withdrawn mood." Jung said he liked it "because it has something that none of the other portraits have," but he predicted that other people would not like it.

Barbara quickly made a place for herself in Jung's inner circle. The fact that she was the first person to come to Jung from reading all of his books gave her a certain distinction and earned her admission to Jung's English seminars in the exclusive Psychological Club, which was restricted to Jung's friends and colleagues. Jung lectured at the club once a week from 1928 to 1939. About a decade later, Barbara started lecturing there, usually once a year. Barbara was not permitted to attend Jung's lectures in German until 1931 because it took her that long to convince those in charge that she could understand German.

Jung once auctioned off an hour of his time at a club auction. He bid for it himself until it went over one hundred francs and then he let someone else have it. That is how he valued time.

Her knowledge of German, as well as of English and French, made her useful to Jung as an editor and translator. She worked with Richard Hull, translator of Jung's *Collected Works,* and she always went through Jung's English writings with him.

Barbara attended all of Jung's lectures, whether in Basel, Einsiedeln, London, Berlin, Ascona, or wherever. Because of her exceptional skill in driving automobiles, she was often elected to drive Jung and others to professional meetings.

In Jung's later years, she had the honor of driving him on Saturday morning pleasure drives.

After one drive, when Jung invited Barbara to eat with him, she was reluctant to tell him that she was tired. Afterward he rebuked her, saying, "I knew that you were tired, but you didn't say so. I need your weaknesses as well as your strengths."

There are advantages and disadvantages to deafness, but the former outweigh the latter.

Barbara's last drive with Jung was exactly one month before his death. She was beginning to suffer some deafness, and he was also having hearing problems, so they had some difficulty communicating. He said to her: "You should not have come today. I have nothing to tell you, and you have had a very dull drive." When he started to repeat this statement as he left the car, Barbara said, "Now look here. Being with you is like being with the sun when it shines. You never had any illusions in your life, and you had better not start now." Jung laughed and got out of the car. That was her last conversation with him. She had a rather ominous feeling about that drive because it was interrupted three times by wedding processions. She could not help thinking of the *Todeshochzeit*, the wedding of death in German mythology, but she kept these fears to herself.

THE INSTITUTE

By 1947 an increasing number of English and American students were coming to Zürich to study, but there were no English seminars available after the war. At a general meeting of the Psychological Club, the committee of the club proposed offering lectures in English. At a second meeting called to consider the proposal, Jung "amazed" the group by his unexpected proposal to found an institute. Realizing how

Jung came to America to lecture but left his shadow behind. He had a wonderful time, but he paid for it.

Barbara Hannah was in a group with Jung and his wife one night. Later Miss Hannah said to him, "Your wife was just not here tonight." Jung replied, "No, she was off with her animus, but she'll come back."

The animus puts a sexual connotation into innocent or meaningful relationships.

The animus tried to keep me from a good night's sleep, so I told the Queen of the Night to take care of this gentleman. She did and I slept all night.

In one of Jung's seminars he said, "All men are anima possessed and all women are animus possessed." When Barbara Hannah asked if she might quote him on that, Jung said, "Perhaps you had better say that people are like sheep, but when you get closer, you sometimes see that the sheep has turned into a wolf!"

Jung was once asked what attitude one should take to an analysand. He replied, "Don't ask me until you have asked the I Ching; then you can ask me."

strongly Jung had opposed the idea two years earlier, after his seventieth birthday, Barbara asked him why he had changed his mind. His reply was, "They would start one anyway between my death and my funeral, so I think it is better to do so while I can still have some influence on its form and perhaps stop some of its worst mistakes."

The institute was founded in 1948, and Jung was president for the first two years. One day, Barbara said to Jung, "You've founded a church." Jung fumed, "Dammit, you're wrong." The next day he said to her, "Dammit, you're right."

At the insistence of Toni Wolff, Barbara became a regular lecturer at the institute. Her first lectures were on the Brontës. Later, at Jung's request, she lectured regularly on *Aion*, originally available only in German and considered by Jung to be his most misunderstood book. Other favorite lecture topics for Barbara included the ego, the shadow, and various aspects of the animus.

After one of her lectures on the animus, a woman said to Barbara, "I can't relate to your discussion of the negative animus because I don't think I have one." Barbara said at that very moment she saw the animus peeping out from behind the woman's neck, making faces and laughing at the woman.

In 1967, Dr. Franz Riklin, then president of the institute, asked Barbara to give the first Jung memorial lecture at the institute on June 6, the sixth anniversary of Jung's death. Her lecture, entitled "Some Glimpses of the Individuation Process in Jung Himself," was warmly received. She felt honored to have been chosen to deliver the first address in what has become an annual commemoration.

Barbara started taking analysands in 1940 and soon became a popular analyst. Objections arose about her becoming a Training Analyst (an analyst approved for training student analysts) because she did not have a doctorate. Even though Jung wrote to the Curatorium stating that he trusted her work and directing that her hours with analysands be certified as if she were a Training Analyst, the Curatorium did not officially declare her to be a Training Analyst for about ten years. When she finally reported her new status to Jung, he said, "Ha."

A suicide is like a murder—the end result is the same—a corpse.

One of Barbara's analysands told her, at the end of an analytical hour, "I'm so discouraged I'm going to leave here and throw myself into the lake." Barbara, recognizing this remark as coming from the negative animus, said to her, "Before you do that, let me ask you a question." Barbara's response shocked the analysand out of her animus possession and brought her back to reality.

Becoming an analyst was not one of Barbara's early goals. She explained:

> There was a time earlier in my life when I vowed never to be analyzed. Later I thought I would like to be an analyst, and after coming to Zürich, it became more possible. People began to come to me for analysis, and Jung said, "You must accept that." We don't know what changes occur in people's lives as a result of analysis. Jung used to say that he often let an analysand leave, thinking that nothing had happened. Then years later, he would get a letter telling him how that person's life had changed. Sometimes people with whom I have worked will write after a period of years to say, "I didn't understand what you were saying at the time. Now what you said has come through."

Jung told the story about a man who committed a murder and went to Protestant pastors, and they were aghast because they did not want to be accessories to the crime. So he went to a Catholic priest who merely asked, "How many?" The man felt accepted. This is what analysands need—to be accepted.

Barbara's three rules for analysts are: patience, patience, patience. She said, "Most people have a skeleton in the closet, but the analyst must not speculate about it. It always comes out." When asked, at ninety-four years of age, why she continued to see analysands, Barbara said, "They just don't go away!"

LECTURES ABROAD

An astrologer, who was a client of Toni Wolff, told Barbara that she was the epitome of introversion and that it would be useless to fight it. The astrologer discouraged her from even attempting to work with people but said, "As you get older, the world will come to you."

Barbara's type, verified by Jung, was introverted intuition with feeling as her auxiliary function and sensation as her inferior function. However, her sensation function always worked well with horses, as well as in finding her way.

Jung said the extravert flies over Mt. Everest, drops a bottle of wine, and thinks he has been there.

The astrologer was wrong when she said that it would be useless for Barbara to fight her introversion. She "fought" it so effectively that by the time she was sixty, some people wondered why she had ever considered herself an introvert.

However, the astrologer was right on one point—the world *did* come to her. More people wanted to be analyzed by her than she could accommodate, and requests for lectures came from Switzerland, England, and America.

In 1952, when Barbara was sixty, she was invited to lecture in New York, Los Angeles, San Francisco, and Philadelphia. Jung urged Barbara to accept the invitation but insisted that she travel by boat. He felt that air travel resulted in leaving bits of one's soul behind.

Barbara bought a new suit for the trip but forgot to wear it. When she stopped in a restaurant in Basel on the way to the port, she discovered that she had on her cleaning clothes! She sent someone back in a taxi to get her new suit. Jung said it was no wonder her lecture tour was such a success—she went to America in her nightgown!

On March 19, 1952, she gave a lecture in New York on active imagination, which was reviewed in the *Bulletin of the Analytical Psychology Club of New York.* An excerpt from the review describes Miss Hannah's lecturing style:

> Miss Hannah disclosed a brilliant, stirring personality. It seemed to many of us that in her delivery and the presentation of her material she showed much of the quality characteristic of Dr. Jung in his seminars. This impression was enhanced by her salty language and her infectious gayety. Her talent for bringing to life the figures of the unconscious was amazing. . . . As an audience our club paid Miss Hannah the tribute of concentrated attention and her words have echoed in many discussions.[2]

Asked about her impressions of America, Barbara said that she was troubled by some of the things she saw there. When she shared her impressions with Jung, he said, "Some of them have given up Jungian psychology and have taken up prestige psychology instead." She explained that prestige psychology is "trying to make a mark for yourself."

In 1968 Barbara and Dr. Franz Riklin were invited to the United States to speak at the second Bailey Island Conference in Maine, celebrating the eightieth birthday of Esther Harding. Given the opportunity to speak on the subject of her choice, she wanted to speak on the beyond but was not sure how to approach

---

[2]"Review of Barbara Hannah's Lecture," *Bulletin of the Analytical Psychology Club of New York* (1952).

it. Then in active imagination she was told, "Yes, you must do it, but get a text to help you. Don't just talk about the beyond or you will be talking nonsense." She found her text in Richard Wilhelm's paper, "Death and Renewal," which discusses Buddhism, Confucianism, and Taoism. Her presentation met with the totally unexpected response of a standing ovation of several minutes.

RELATIONSHIP WITH MARIE-LOUISE VON FRANZ

The story of Barbara Hannah would not be complete without reporting her relationship with Dr. Marie-Louise von Franz. The two women met for the first time in 1937 when they were both involved in a translation project for Jung.

The record is not clear on whether their decision to share living quarters was the result of a dream or a suggestion from Jung. In any case, Jung was pleased with the arrangement, which on the surface seemed to be an unlikely one in view of the age difference. Barbara was forty-six and Marie-Louise was twenty-three. When Barbara asked Jung, "Why are you so keen on putting us together?" Jung replied:

> She has a very negative mother complex, and I want her to see that not all women are such brutes as her mother. It will also teach you not to be jealous, and you had better not be jealous of her because she is a genius. [Jung said that Dr. von Franz was the only one of his pupils who fully understood his ideas.] The real reason you should live together is that your chief interest will be analysis and analysts should not live alone. They get too much into their patients' material, and it is better for them to have some difficulties of their own. I have

> given you someone who will give you a lot of trouble.

Jung's perception was correct. Barbara recalled that neither of them liked living with the other at first. She said that they "fought the good fight" for ten years and nearly parted. Jung had promised them that he would be available to them when they found the other difficult, but unfortunately, he had a heart attack two days after they moved in together, so they had to "fight their own battles" for a few months. After the first ten years, "we hardly had a row," Barbara said. They were a strong support for each other when Jung died. "I don't know if either of us could have stood his death had we lived alone," she said.

At Jung's funeral, there was a violent storm during the service and Ruth Bailey said, "That's Jung saying to the preacher, 'Can't you stop?' "

Barbara and Marie-Louise lived in a flat on the Zürichsee until they moved to the house at Lindenbergstrasse 15, which they shared until Barbara's death some twenty-five years later. In 1958, Marie-Louise built the Tower on a hill above Bollingen which served as a retreat for both her and Barbara. Barbara wrote most of her biography of Jung at the Tower.

The unconscious often dredges up the most fiendish dreams just before a holiday; it seems to take a delight in making one work before a vacation.

When asked, "What makes Barbara Hannah such a unique person?" Dr. von Franz responded:

> The straightforwardness and honesty of her character. She has been a loyal friend through all these years. The women around Jung had a jealousy problem, and naturally, we also had one, but she was not catty about it. You could have it out with her, which you could not do with many people.
>
> She helped me by preventing me from making childish scenes. She was more grown-up; I was nineteen when I began my analysis with Jung. I was inclined to make a childish fuss about things that were of no interest whatso-

> ever to Jung. I could often react with her about those things so that it was not necessary for me to carry them to Jung. She helped me a lot with her common sense. She is a model of the individuation process.

In response to the question, "Have you often dreamed of her?" Dr. von Franz replied with a gleam, "Oh, yes, in all colors! In the beginning, I projected my negative mother onto her, because she could be my mother since she is twenty-three years older. I do not dream of her so often now, but when I do, she appears as a benevolent companion and a loyal friend."

Barbara Hannah spoke of Dr. von Franz with the greatest professional admiration and with personal affection. Good-natured bantering characterized their relationship. When Barbara was ninety-two, she cancelled an afternoon appointment because she was too tired after spending the morning with the hairdresser and the manicurist. When Dr. von Franz learned of the cancellation, she said to Barbara, "At your age you should not be so vain!"

They both had international reputations as analysts and writers.

CREATIVE DAIMON

"Writing was a thing I did to keep myself alive," Barbara said, "and to keep myself in Jungian psychology." She published her first book, *Striving Toward Wholeness,* when she was eighty. The book was the outgrowth of her lectures on the Brontës and is concerned with the individuation process in literature. She said she felt a great longing to write the book. While she was pondering the difficulty of dealing with the subject, "the image of the Garden of Eden presented itself . . . as the connecting thread."[3] Although she discussed the book with Jung and wrote three chapters while he was living, the book was not published until after his death.

The story of Barbara Hannah's life could accurately be entitled, "Striving Toward Wholeness." Long before she became interested in psychology, she was attracted to wholeness, to people without affectation who were close to nature. She explained: "I loved to draw peasants, people who had been on the soil and were whole. I wouldn't draw anything unless it had something of wholeness."

When asked to define wholeness, Barbara said, "It is one of the things you don't speak about." But in her book she writes:

> In every living creature the urge for its own totality is perhaps the strongest and most fundamental of all urges. . . . We have largely forgotten that our first obligation, after all, is to be a simple human being, and that the simple human being has a certain quality of wholeness.[4]

Originally Barbara expressed her idea of wholeness through her art but later she followed Jung's example of helping people to make their lives whole. After two hours with Jung, "I knew that he was the only whole person I had ever seen," she said. "To be whole instead of perfect is perhaps Jung's greatest idea."

Her second book and her favorite was *Jung, His Life and Work: A Biographical Memoir.* Although when she came to Zürich, Barbara had no reason to expect that she would be one

---

[3]Barbara Hannah, *Striving Toward Wholeness* (New York: G. P. Putnam's Sons, 1971), p. ix.

[4]Hannah, *Striving,* pp. 4–5.

of Jung's biographers, she knew from the beginning that she was in the presence of greatness. She kept careful notes on her conversations and analytical hours with Jung, as well as on his lectures and seminars. (She missed only two seminars in all those years.) In the preface to the biography, she disclaims that the book is a definitive biography, yet a reviewer calls it "a biography lover's dream."[5] "I tell the story as I knew him, just as I saw him," she said. And she was one of the few who knew Jung well.

Barbara Hannah wrote the biography of Jung at the request of the C. G. Jung Foundation in New York, on the recommendation of Esther Harding, who considered her the most qualified person. When Vernon Brooks and William Kennedy first approached her about writing the book, she was somewhat reluctant but a subsequent dream convinced her. In the dream, she was in the beyond when someone told her, "Go back and write everything you know about the beyond." She reasoned that Jung was in the beyond and that everything she knew about the beyond came from him. Although the message was indirect, she considered it to be a "go-ahead" signal from the unconscious.

In the preface to the book, Barbara writes:

> In *Memories, Dreams, Reflections* Jung wrote almost entirely of his inner life, which was far more meaningful than any outer event. It was also of this inner side of his life that he almost always talked to me. I have tried to follow the course of his life chronologically, showing how he first lived his psychology and only much later formulated in words what he had lived.[6]

---

[5]Barbara Hoffman, "Review of *Jung, His Life and Work: A Biographical Memoir*, by Barbara Hannah," *Best Sellers* (March 1977), p. 393.

[6]Barbara Hannah, *Jung, His Life and Work: A Biographical Memoir* (New York: G. P. Putnam's Sons, 1976), Preface.

Barbara's third book, *Encounters with the Soul: Active Imagination*, was the culmination of a lifetime of work with what Marie-Louise von Franz called "the most powerful tool in Jungian psychology for achieving wholeness."[7] In her book, Barbara says, "Perhaps the simplest definition of active imagination is to say that it gives us the opportunity of opening negotiations, and in time, coming to terms with these forces or figures in the unconscious."[8]

Jung told a man to do active imagination. The man asked if he could have his wife there and also listen to the radio.

When Barbara first learned of active imagination and tried to use it in her work with Toni Wolff and Peter Baynes, she had little success but still attempted to work with it. After she started to work with Jung, he taught her the secret of it so that it became very meaningful. She discovered that she had to go as deep as possible to really get at the truth imbedded in the unconscious. She said that she learned a lot about active imagination from reading *The Secret of the Golden Flower* which was published the year after she came to Zürich.

Jung explained to a group of doctors what he did in active imagination. He was up on a mountain and there was a cloud a mile long. He talked to her (the German word for cloud is feminine) and found her very meaningful. He asked if he could take her home. He put the cloud on his head and went home but he could not get inside the door. He was stuck there for three days. Then he asked the cloud, "Are you my fantasy?" Immediately the cloud collapsed so he could put it in his pocket, and the problem was solved.

Toward the end of his life, Jung told Barbara:

> People have understood passive imagination, but only a few have understood what active imagination really is. Passive imagination is used in every hospital when people are encouraged to draw or sculpt, but active imagination is something else. You are actually in it yourself, and people don't understand that the figures in active imagination are real, psychologically real. Of course, it cannot be rationally proved.

At ninety-three, Barbara said, "Sometimes I think I don't understand it because you hear

---

[7]Hannah, *Encounters*, p. 2.

[8]Ibid., p. 16.

things that are surprising. At first you think you are making up things, but you have to accept whatever comes. That is not easy because the unconscious tells us things we do not know and often do not want to hear." However, in her book, she explains:

> If we honestly want to find our own wholeness, to live our own individual fate as fully as possible, if we truly want to abolish illusion on principle and find the truth of our own inner being, however little we like to be the way we are, then there is nothing that can help us so much in our endeavour as active imagination.[9]

ON RELIGION

There is something divine about doubt which keeps you struggling. The gift of doubt is often the crown of life.

Barbara Hannah recalled a statement of Jung to the effect that "we have found a new way to live. Some people think we have found it in analytical psychology. I wish I agreed with them because then I could give my mind to something else, but I don't agree, so I go on searching."

Barbara Hannah became disillusioned with institutional religion at an early age. However, her religious upbringing left its imprint on her; there was something of a vacuum in her life until she went to Zürich and found the answer in analytical psychology. Barbara explained: "I had completely lost my religion when I came to Zürich, but I learned once more to believe in God and prayer. They were all gone but they came back after I learned the true side of them with Jung." She said that "thy will be done" was the one thing she retained from her early religious training. "I always realized that one didn't know enough to live by one's own will." She explained that if she had known enough psychology, she would have realized that the "ego has to give in to the Self." Essentially, she

---

[9]Ibid., p. 12.

equates God with the Self, and like the Self, her God has both a dark and a light side.

Barbara's philosophy was greatly influenced by Meister Johann Eckhart (1260–1328), a German Dominican mystic whom Barbara did not consider a mystic. "He's much more practical than most mystics," she said. Barbara also thought that it was nonsense that Jung was called a mystic. "He was no more mystical than the cat," she declared.

Barbara said that if we recognize the importance of the infinite, which we really cannot define, then we are not so given to frivolities and to wasting our lives. She quoted Jung as saying that life is only worth living if you realize that you have something of the infinite in you and you try to live that piece of the infinite.

Jung's father took him to Vitznau one day, but there was only enough money to pay for one ticket to the top of the Rigi. Jung went and had a vision of God on top of the mountain, but he also had fun. Later he commented, "One does not preclude the other."

We have two thousand years of Christian experience in our life stream.

Under all our desires is the desire for the infinite.

VOICES FROM THE UNCONSCIOUS

When Barbara was ninety-three, she said, "I didn't listen well enough to the unconscious; that is why I have had to live such a long time." People who have worked with her probably would not agree that she did not listen well. Many are indebted to her for making them aware of the reality of the unconscious. She explained her approach to analysands in this way: "I do my best to focus their attention on the reality of the unconscious until I feel that they know from experience that they are dealing with something which is just as real as the outside world."[10]

The unconscious tried to make itself known to Barbara at an early age, even though she did not recognize it at the time. A recurring dream from her childhood bothered her terribly:

In the film Face to Face, *an opening scene shows Jung throwing bread into the lake for the swans and ducks before going into the house. Barbara Hannah asked Jung, "Did you think of the symbolic meaning of that—spreading bread on the surface of the unconscious—so that those who wished to eat could do so and the others would disregard it?" Jung said, "No, I hadn't thought of that; the unconscious must have arranged it."*

[10]Ibid., p. 13.

I was standing at the gate of the House of Commons in London, and there was a revolution going on outside. I was always told that if I walked out into the revolution, it would stop. Then there was another version where I was in a little cart and was taken to be hanged.

Fowler McCormick was traveling with Jung in India, and Jung told him a dream. Fowler made some foolish remark about the dream, and Jung said it was that comment which put him on the track of understanding it.

The dream was so frightening that she was reluctant to go to sleep for fear that she would dream it again. It was the only childhood dream that she remembered, and she never understood it until many years later when she told it to Jung. He explained: "You see, you've got to accept the opposites. If you do it voluntarily, things will turn out well. If you refuse to do it, you'll be hung between the opposites, because it is your fate to accept them."

THOUGHTS ON OLD AGE AND DEATH

Barbara seemed to consider old age more of a discipline than a blessing. "I left something undone," she said early in 1985, "and had to live ninety-three years to do it. The greatest thing is to do it younger because living to ninety-three really isn't fun." Nevertheless, she felt that she was kept alive for a purpose—to do something—and that gave meaning to her life.

It is better to have a basket full of scorpions than to have an empty basket.

"I now feel certain things will be told to me only because I'm so old," she said. However, she protested being considered the archetype of the "wise old woman." In her youth, an older friend told her that as we get older, we lose the desire to be remembered. At ninety-three, she said she was at the place where she did not care whether or not she is remembered. The fact that she knew Jung well is the only thing worth remembering, she said.

A dream in 1985 provided her with serenity and a sense of adventure in her old age:

> *Jung and I were riding horses on a battlefield with bombs and shells dropping all around us. Although the situation was fraught with danger, I thought: "I'm not in the least bit afraid. So long as I keep my horse's nose close to the tail of Jung's horse, I'll be quite safe."*

In a very real sense, Barbara Hannah kept close to Jung, not only in his lifetime, but also after his death. Six weeks after he died, he appeared to her in active imagination and said, "I haven't gone, I shall be just the same as before." She said that death did not separate her from Jung. "I can't see him, but I can still talk with him," she said. "Jung is a spirit presence; often it seems that he has not left. The years since his death have been meaningful, even though he's not here."

In his later years Jung liked to talk about death. Once when Jung and Barbara were sitting on a bench in the mountains, Barbara asked Jung what death would be like. Jung replied, "We are sitting here today and after I am gone, we will still be sitting here." Barbara used to impress on her analysands over sixty the need for facing the fact of death realistically. Jung asked if she didn't think she should lower the age level.

Barbara said that the only thing she was sure of about life after death was that we will get out of time and space. She speculated that we will not have bodies and wondered what that would be like. "I have some other ideas of how it will be, but they are not worth anything because they cannot be proved."

When she was interviewed at ninety-three, she said that she wanted to use her remaining time to reread some of Jung's books, especially *Psychology and Alchemy*, *Mysterium Coniunctionis*, and *Aion*, three of his books which she did not know well enough, she said. She read *Memories*,

Jung once said he thought he was dead—but he reasoned that if he were, he could walk through the wall. He tried it and couldn't so he knew he was not dead.

Jung had a vision of a friend who had died. In the vision, the figure of his friend beckoned to him and Jung thought, "If I refuse him, that will really be discourteous because he was my friend." So he followed him into the library, and his friend pointed to four red books on the top shelf and drew attention to the second book. The next day Jung inquired of the man's widow if he might see her library. Sure enough, there were four red books on the top shelf and the second one was titled The Legacy of the Dead.

After writing Mysterium Coniunctionis, *Jung said he really didn't understand it himself; he just pushed back the horizons a little.*

Dreams, Reflections least fifty times and in her ninety-third year she read *Answer to Job* eight times. Jung said that *Answer to Job* was the only one of his books in which he would not change so much as a comma. "If Jung set such a value on *Answer to Job*, I should know it by heart," she said.

When asked what three wishes she would like to have granted, she was willing to settle for two: to be rid of her laziness and to understand the unconscious better.

When death came to Barbara Hannah on September 4, 1986, it came as a fulfillment of those words with which she ended her Bailey Island lecture on "The Beyond":

> Only by detachment—that quality which Meister Eckhart values higher than any other—can we "form a conception of life after death or create some image of it." But we can only afford this detachment by the utmost attachment to life and by a determination to live it as faithfully as possible, till we really come to the right time for, what the Chinese call, the greatest good fortune of all: namely finding our own specific death, which will crown and not tear apart our life.[11]

We influence the world most through what we are, not what we say.

So what is the myth of this extraordinary woman, who had no academic degrees, yet was an internationally known analyst and author? "Before I came to Zürich," she said, "I had not been getting along at all; I lived a rather ordinary life." But her meeting with Jung, and her years of association with him and his ideas, made the difference. Barbara's attraction to Jung from his books is inexplicable, but although she

---

[11]Barbara Hannah, "The Beyond," Bailey Island Lecture, (Maine, 1962).

recognized his genius from reading his books, she said, "His books are nothing compared with him. Now I have met a man who knows everything. He is fully a man in every way. Here is a person who will never let me down. Life will never be the same." She found in Jung an ideal whose luster was never dimmed by years of close association.

Those who knew Barbara Hannah best agree that she clearly validated Jung's ideas by achieving the individuation that Jung considered the ultimate goal of life. She achieved this state by marching to her "drummer," and her drummer was the unconscious.

REFLECTIONS AFTER THE DEATH OF BARBARA HANNAH

by Dean L. Frantz

I had planned to see Miss Hannah in August 1986 to get her final approval of my manuscript but the scheduled visit was postponed because she had not finished reading it. My uneasy feeling about the change in plans was confirmed when I received a call informing me that Barbara Hannah had slipped into the beyond that morning.

Barbara Hannah dead? Impossible! No more face-to-face talks, no letters granting me the privilege of talking with her, no more encouragement from this woman who for me was the living epitome of Jung's psychology?

But as the reality of her departure from this world became clear, I reflected on the privilege I enjoyed of knowing her for almost two decades, beginning in 1967.

When I arrived at Miss Hannah's house in Küsnacht for my first appointment, I rang the bell with considerable trepidation and was admitted by a woman who looked like a Swiss peasant. I was shown upstairs, where I was greeted by Miss Hannah, a woman with regal bearing, snow white hair, delicately carved features, and penetrating eyes. She shook my hand and invited me to be seated. She sat with her legs outstretched on an ottoman, and I realized that she was rather tall for a woman. Our chairs nearly touched, creating at once an atmosphere of intimacy and rapport.

On a little round table in front of Miss Hannah were some scattered papers, a brass Buddha, and a vase of fresh flowers. In my hundreds of appointments with her, I never saw her table without fresh flowers. Two bookcases lined the walls, and although my intuition told me that the wisdom of the ages was there, somehow this accumulated wisdom seemed to be incarnated in Miss Hannah, sharing her warmth and insight with a neophyte in Jungian psychology.

Another aspect of her consulting room intrigued me. There was a telephone on a low stand by her chair. When the phone rang and the caller wished to speak to Dr. Marie-Louise von Franz, Miss Hannah would grab a large bell, walk to the stairway leading to the first floor, and vigorously ring the bell until Dr. von Franz picked up the phone. The telephone ritual was one I witnessed dozens of times in my years of analysis. When Miss Hannah was especially annoyed by the interference of a call, she would often mutter to herself, "There's that damn phone again."

I sensed that Miss Hannah knew how to ask the right questions—firmly but not ruthlessly. My bonding with her was immediate. I knew that no secrets could be withheld from her, but I also sensed a warm compassion for my years as a professional in religious vocations. In that first hour, I heard "All haste is of the devil," a phrase I was to hear often during the next few years, and "vocatus atque non vocatus deus aderit" (Invited or not, God will be there), the words carved in stone at Bollingen and also carved over the door of Jung's house in Küsnacht.

My first hour with Miss Hannah passed all too quickly, but in that short time she had plumbed the depths of my soul. I felt as if I had known this truly "wise old woman" for a lifetime. When I left that upper room for the first time, I did not know what the future held for me, but I realized that life would never be the same.

Two years after that first meeting, I took a leave of absence from my position with a liberal arts college and returned to Zürich for the summer. I had the good fortune to work with Miss Hannah and also with Dr. Riklin, then president of the Jung Institute. Working with these two was an unforgettable experience, tempered by the untimely death of Dr. Riklin in mid-summer. His death was a personal loss to both Miss Hannah and me.

I was fascinated by this brief exposure to Jungian psychology, but seeing no chance of going further, I returned to my work at the college. Two years later I went to Zürich again to work with Miss Hannah and to share with her some of my dreams. Her comments were very pointed: "The years between fifty and seventy are the most important in life. Don't waste them. Fund-raising is killing your soul. If you continue in your present job, you are going to lose your soul."

A year later when I resigned my college position to begin my studies at the Institute, Miss Hannah wrote: "I congratulate you on your courage in making your momentous decision and only hope you find it as rewarding as I did when I made mine to come here." When I accepted the academic position, I had intended to spend the rest of my professional life at this college in the cornfields of Indiana.

During my four years as a student in Zürich, I never missed an appointment, nor was I late. Not that I always went eagerly, because my dreams and my intuition often warned me about what awaited me. But I also knew that once having started the journey, there was no turning back. Miss Hannah made it clear from the start that a great deal of pain was inevitable because she knew from her own experience the suffering which is the lot of those who make the inner journey. At eighty-three, she said to me, "I have known Jung's ideas for forty years and I still suffer enormously at times." This personal testimony was another way of emphasizing what I often heard from her: "The achievement of consciousness always involves suffering—*always*."

Miss Hannah did not spare her analysands because, as she once said, "If people are nicey-nice to each other, there will be hell to pay the next day." When the situation demanded plain talk, she could deliver. If people did not live up to what she regarded as their potential, she minced no words. She had only scathing comments for a woman who read her husband's dreams and active imagination, and she made sharp remarks about people whom she felt had betrayed the essential core of Jung's concepts. She once described a person as "playing third violin in a second-rate orchestra."

But she could be just as critical of herself as of others. When she realized that she had been the victim of an animus attack, she said, "There's that damned animus again; I thought I had taken care of him. . . ." When I was reluctant to do what my dreams demanded of me, she said without equivocation, "If you don't do what your unconscious is clearly asking you to do, you are going to be in trouble with me." Then she added this clincher, "The door has clanged shut behind you."

Miss Hannah's trust in and obedience to the unconscious was total. She once said to me, "I didn't know how to get you moving without shocking you, but your unconscious has taken over and given impetus and direction to your analysis." I once commented to her that "life would have been simpler if. . . ." To which she dryly remarked, "Of course, life would have been simpler. Vegetable life is always simpler than human life, but who wants to be a vegetable?" When I was pondering a decision at a critical juncture of my analysis, she brought me back to reality with, "Why do you insist on making a premature judgment when you don't even know what the unconscious says?" Early in my analysis I learned the truth of the statement: "The unconscious is like the sea—throw yourself into it and you will drown, but trust it and it will buoy you up."

Her whimsical attitude brightened many a day. Once when I said to her, "I would not have wanted to miss a single day of my life," she remarked, "I could have missed a few at the beginning, but not during the last forty-four years." Often she would search for a missing book or paper and, not finding it, would mutter, "Strange things are happening around here; things just dematerialize," or, "The devil must have put his paws on it."

One of the familiar sights around Küsnacht and Zürich was Barbara Hannah driving her little English car to her appointments, a privilege she did not relinquish until she was almost ninety. Her nephew once told her about a man in a quarry who thought all spinsters were dull and unfulfilled. Her nephew told the man that he had an aunt who certainly did not fit that description. To which the man replied, "Then she must have cheated." That man obviously did not know Barbara Hannah.

Other memories surfaced as I realized that Miss Hannah was no longer in the land of the living: her visit to our home in Meilen; her introduction of Peter Birkhauser to me when I was searching for a thesis subject; my driving her to Basel one day to visit Peter in his studio and her heated exchange with him because she disagreed with one of his paintings; visits to the Tower where she and Dr. von Franz cooked meals in their fireplace; her sharing with me relevant chapters of her biography of Jung before its publication; her service on my thesis committee with the understanding that I should not expect easy approval just because she was my analyst; her frequent references to the Bible and to the writings of Meister Eckhart; her patience in putting up with my pastor's persona because she too had come from a parish setting.

Her correspondence with me over a period of twenty years reveals some choice insights into Miss Hannah. In a letter from the Tower after a late spring snow, she wrote, "D--n this snow, I hate snow." In another letter she reported that when she and Dr. von Franz returned from a trip to England and found the furnace not working in their Küsnacht house, they went to the Tower at Bollingen. Miss Hannah wrote, "Thankfully we came here where there are no modern gadgets." In a letter to me while I was spending a few months in Indiana she wrote, "I hope you are escaping the ecclesiastical snares of America."

But the memory of Miss Hannah that I treasure most is of that time midway through my studies at the Institute when my meager financial resources had long since vanished. I was in the "depths of despair" and saw no alternative to leaving my studies and returning to the States. Then Miss Hannah said, "You are not going to leave before receiving your diploma, I have a plan to get you the money." She arranged for me to borrow the necessary money from her, with the stipulation that I repay it after establishing my practice.

Had it not been for Miss Hannah, I would not be where I am today. But the real debt I owe her can never be repaid. Often as I struggle to help people find their way through the maze of life's problems, some word of hers will appear to shed light on the situation, or some story about Jung that she shared with me will illumine an aspect that had escaped me.

I would be less than honest were I to say that I enjoyed those years of intensive, soul-searching, sometimes heartrending analysis with Miss Hannah. There were days when I thought I must be the greatest fool in the world to spend good money to be tortured in this manner. But there were other days when I sensed that she was my guide and companion on a journey toward a kind of wholeness that I had never known. I also realized that to give up was to risk losing my soul, as she predicted. However, without her support and encouragement, I would have quit long before the finish.

Obviously, Miss Hannah's work with analysands was an important part of her life. But her published works have preserved for us many insights of Jung that otherwise would have been lost. Thus her life has reached far beyond the confines of those who knew her personally.

Her death brought to me a genuine sense of loss. But I realize that my life has been greatly enriched by knowing this remarkable person who truly deserves to be called a wise old woman.

She is gone from our midst, but she continues to inspire us by her example of wholeness and by her published works. She will be remembered as one of the persons who knew Jung best, as one who was able to transmit to future generations, in words that could be understood, the essential core of Jung's psychology, which speaks to the souls of individuals everywhere.

INTRODUCTION TO "THE BEYOND"

Dr. W. R. Sanford is a Jungian analyst in Del Mar, California, and offers the following memory of Barbara Hannah's lecture at Bailey Island on the occasion of Esther Harding's birthday in 1968.

In 1962 I had an analytical hour with Max Zeller. As I went to leave, he asked, "You are going to Bailey Island, aren't you?" I replied, "Where's that—I never heard of it." Zeller responded, "You should attend this conference, it's going to be great." My answer was "I have just returned from the first long vacation I have ever taken in my professional life, and I can't possibly do that." Zeller replied, "I think you will be sorry if you don't go."

I drove home and had a dream that night. In my dream I went to my office and opened the closet door to hang up my coat. There was a box on the floor, like an old apple box. My curiosity led me to open the lid and to my astonishment, it was filled to the brim with money! Within thirty minutes I called New York to see if they would accept my late registration, and I called an airline for plane reservations. Both responses were in the affirmative, and within a week I was on my way to Bailey Island.

The second Bailey Island conference in 1962 was held in honor of Esther Harding's eightieth birthday. It was attended by about two hundred people, thirty-two of whom had attended the first Bailey Island conference. I will never forget Miss Hannah's lecture, "The Beyond." When she stood up to speak, she picked up the microphone and said, "I noticed yesterday that this thing is rather temperamental, and I'm not sure if it's going to like me." The chairman suggested that she stand a bit closer to the microphone; then she read a sentence, to which he replied, "That's good." She responded, "I noticed yesterday that at times your voice was too good for it." Her remark brought a hearty laugh from the audience. Her lecture was outstanding. Afterwards, she received enormous applause and a standing ovation which lasted several minutes.

The Beyond

It is, of course, quite impossible for me to say anything in the least definite about the subject I have had the foolhardiness to choose as my theme today. But two special things urged me to do so, beyond and above the natural interest in the subject that grows on one more and more in old age.

The first is to be found in *Memories, Dreams, Reflections* where Jung says: "A man should be able to say he has done his best to form a conception of life after death, or to create some image of it—even if he must confess his failure. Not to have done so is a vital loss. For the question that is posed to him is the age-old heritage of humanity: an archetype rich in secret life, which seeks to add itself to our own individual life in order to make it whole."[1]

And the second compelling reason was in a dream of my own. About two years ago I dreamed that I had passed through a door numbered 3 or 9. There was a numinous feeling, and I was slowly wondering if this was death, when I was told to go back through the same door, because I had permission to return to the earth in order to write down all I knew about the life beyond death, as if I had been for a short time in that world.

The very evening after I had the dream, we dined with Mr. Kennedy and Mr. Brooks and the former suggested a subject for a further book. The synchronicity of the dream and the outer event made me take up Mr. Kennedy's suggestion, but the fact that, taken more literally, the dream said I should write all I knew about the Beyond itself—combined with the just quoted passage from Jung—has never quite left me in peace, so that, when Marie-Louise von Franz suggested I should take up this theme for Dr. Harding's birthday, I knew at once that I must make the attempt, even if I must only confess my failure.

But—as is usually my custom when confronted with an especially

---

This lecture was given at the Second Bailey Island Conference held in honor of Dr. Esther Harding's eightieth birthday in August 1968. A copy appeared in *Quadrant* (Winter 1969). This version is based on Barbara Hannah's own manuscript.

[1]C. G. Jung, *Memories, Dreams, Reflections* (New York: Pantheon Books, 1961), p. 302.

difficult task—I took up the subject in active imagination and was told I should certainly try but only if I could find a material as a basis for what I said. I thought over many materials but none even began to satisfy me except a paper on "Death and Renewal in China," by Richard Wilhelm, which Marie-Louise von Franz had given me to read some years before.[2] As she gives the most relevant part in her new book on numbers, I felt reluctant to use it but, with her generous encouragement, I at last overcame my misgivings. I must also thank her here for her patience in listening to my difficulties in writing this paper and for many valuable suggestions.

The paper in question is not an old Chinese text but rather Wilhelm's own summing up of the Chinese point of view on death and renewal seen from more than one side. The most important point of all seems to be held in common by their three chief religions—Taoism, Confucianism, and Buddhism; but I must own to my surprise, of all these three, Confucianism seems much the nearest to our own Western point of view. This is really because, as is well known, Buddhism is concerned with a long series of incarnations, which culminate in the goal of Nirvana, an achievement where the individual has at last fulfilled all his karma and may dissolve forever in an eternal impersonal bliss. The Taoists also seem little concerned with the ultimate fate of the individual or with how long he survives, but the Confucians put a much higher value on consciousness and on this human life altogether and thus indirectly on individual survival in the Beyond.

As is well known, the Chinese—in fact, the whole East—have a very different attitude to the opposites than we have in the West. It is amazing how passionately—even after many decades of studying Jung—many of us still cling to the white opposite and condemn the black. In this age, indeed, there seem to be quite as many or even more people who find the black opposite the most rewarding, but they thus as a rule carefully avoid the moral problem—that Jung always said was indispensable—and thus prevent themselves from realizing that they are repressing the white opposite. And as Jung frequently pointed out, it is not pursuing perfection but holding the balance between both opposites that is the vital thing now. In "Late Thoughts" in his *Memories*, for instance, he points out that "Evil has become a determinent reality. . . . We must learn to handle it, since it is here to stay. How we can live with it without horrible consequences cannot for the present be conceived."[3]

---

[2]Richard Wilhelm, "Death and Renewal in China,"

[3]Jung, *Memories*, p. 328.

And he continues: "Touching evil brings with it the grave peril of succumbing to it. We must, therefore, no longer succumb to anything at all, not even to good. A so-called good to which we succumb loses its ethical character. Not that there is anything bad in it on that score, but evil results develop because one has succumbed to it.[4] Every form of addiction is bad, no matter whether the narcotic be alcohol, or morphine or idealism. . . . Recognition of the reality of evil necessarily relativizes the good, and the evil likewise, converting both into halves of a paradoxical whole."[5]

I have just reminded you of how Jung himself regarded the opposites, because it leads the way into the whole Chinese philosophy of life which – in contrast to the West – is all based on the equality of the opposites. Those of us who use the I Ching are well acquainted with the equal opposites of Yang and Yin, masculine and feminine, but perhaps we are less aware that Chinese philosophy regards life and death also as a pair of equal opposites on which all human beings are based. In fact, if it tends to favor one of those opposites, it is rather death. Wilhelm points out that the Chinese simply do not prize life as we do; we rate it so much higher than death. On the contrary, they do not regard life as quite real but more as a temporary illusion, so clearly it is easier and more natural for them to hold the balance between life and death than it is for us. Some of the oldest documents in China point out that the greatest good fortune that a man can meet is to find a death that crowns his life, his own specific death, and the greatest misfortune that threatens him is to find an untimely death that tears his life apart instead of completing it. Therefore the ancient sages in China absolutely refused to call any man happy till after his death.

As death is valued so highly in China, it is natural that the Chinese also regard fear of death as a great stumbling block and that one of the most important tasks of a well-spent life is to educate oneself in fearlessness towards death, a fearlessness, Wilhelm emphasizes, that is ready to look at all that befalls us in the face and is anxious to come to terms with everything that the future could bring. Therefore they spend a great deal of time – already in life – in thinking about death; in fact, they fulfill the task that Jung advises us to fulfill: they really do their best "to form a conception of life after death or to create some image of it."

Wilhelm tells us a good deal about how they set about this task,

---

[4]The German (p. 331) is "aber es entwickelt bose Folgen, weil man ihm verfallen ist." The English translation (p. 329) "to have succumbed to it may breed trouble" seems to me too mild.

[5]Jung, *Memories*, p. 328–329.

and this is the reason that I felt this paper might give us some hints for our own efforts in this direction. Although, as always when we are dealing with Eastern ideas, we must not forget that any imitation of the East does not agree with Western man, Jung says of this in his introduction to *The Secret of the Golden Flower*: "The Chinese can fall back upon the authority of his entire culture. If he starts on the long way, he does what is recognized as being the best of all the things he could do. But the Westerner who wishes to start upon this way, if he is truly serious about it, has all authority against him. That is why it is infinitely easier for a man to imitate the Chinese way."[6] But "it is sad indeed when the European departs from his own nature and imitates the East or 'affects' it in any way. The possibilities open to him would be so much greater if he would remain true to himself and develop out of his own nature all that the East has brought forth from its inner being in the course of centuries."[7] Keeping this in mind, we will see what hints for our own work we can find in this excellent article of Richard Wilhelm's, although I must emphasize that time forbids me to give you any idea of its rich content; I can only pick out a point here and there.

Wilhelm points out that this "long way," as Jung calls it, requires the most serious and concentrated thinking, but that this is something very different from what we understand by thinking in the West. Chinese thought is far more substantial than ours, an active thinking that even has an effect on the realm of objective existence. To sum up, they would not say "I think" but "it thinks in me," and they explore these objective thoughts as we might explore an unknown territory on earth.

Jung learned this kind of thinking the hard way years before he knew anything of Chinese thought. I first realized how much of the "hard way" it was when he was struggling to find his way in the unknown labyrinth of alchemy. He explained how lost and near despair he often felt and added: "I have experienced nothing like it, since my first confrontation with the unconscious but that was worse, even much worse."

It was in a conversation with the figure he called Philemon that Jung first learned of this different substantial kind of thought. He writes: "He [Philemon] said I treated thoughts as if I generated them myself, but in his view thoughts were like animals in the forest, or people in a room, or birds in the air, and added: 'If you should see

---

[6]Richard Wilhelm, *The Secret of the Golden Flower* (London: Routledge and Kegan Paul, 1931, reprinted 1965, 1967, 1969), p. 95.

[7]Ibid., p. 85.

people in a room, you would not think that you had made those people, or that you were responsible for them.' It was he who taught me psychic objectivity, the reality of the psyche."[8] And exploring the unconscious with this kind of objective thinking eventually led Jung to the basic foundation—that is the same in East and West—of the human psyche, to the foursquare "mandala as an expression of the Self." So that when Wilhelm sent him *The Secret of the Golden Flower* in 1928—more than ten years after his own discoveries—he tells us that it "gave me undreamed of confirmation of my ideas about the mandala and the circumambulation of the center. That was the first event which broke through my isolation. I became aware of an affinity; I could establish ties with something and someone."[9] It was with the kind of thinking, taught to Jung by Philemon, and which he subsequently taught us as active imagination, that the Chinese explore the Beyond and try to form some conception of it.

Wilhelm tells us that the Confucians hold that two opposite principles form two poles between which everything lies. They have many names for these principles of which I will only mention heaven and earth, because they hold that the human being has two souls, one belonging to each, as it were. At death the vegetative soul falls down into the depths of the earth where it then forms part of an ancestral deposit of death and rebirth. This is the reason that every Chinese wants to die in China, or at least be buried in his own soil. But there is another soul which at death soars into the heights. This is the soul which is capable of becoming spiritual already in life. Wilhelm points out that the spirit is not something that grows naturally in man, but something that he must make a great effort to acquire in the course of his life. According to Confucian ideas, this spirit has a kind of consciousness that can survive death. It never dissolves at once, any more than the body, and therefore the Chinese always speak in the death chamber as if the deceased were still present, in order that he may gain time to separate himself from the body.

This is certainly an archetypal idea, lying in the unconscious, which can come to the surface anywhere and at any time. If you will excuse a personal memory: an aunt I had never liked died when I was about seven or eight. Immediately I thought how careful I must be not to say, if possible even to think, anything negative about her, because I took for granted that she would now hear everything I said and even

---

[8]Jung, *Memories*, p. 189.

[9]Ibid., p. 197.

probably what I thought. I instinctively kept this conviction to myself but I was nevertheless amazed years afterwards to learn that, at any rate in my family, it was not a generally recognized fact.

Wilhelm goes on to point out that a dynamic point of view is to be found everywhere in China. They do not emphasize the solidity of matter as we do but rather regard it as a dynamic condition. As the spirit undoubtedly exists but has no substantial existence, it is rather regarded by the Confucians as a tendency towards consciousness:

> It naturally leads a somewhat precarious existence unless it has been so concentrated in the course of life that it has already *built itself a kind of subtle body of a spiritual nature,* made as it were of thoughts and works, a body that gives consciousness a support when it has to leave its former assistant, the body. This psychic body is at first very delicate, so that only the very wisest men can preserve it and find their refuge in it after death.[10]

Ordinary people cannot achieve this, and therefore their existence after death depends on the thoughts of the survivors, which is the underlying meaning of the whole ancestor cult in China.

This striking formulation of the possibility of building a subtle body during our lifetime, which would afford us the same refuge and home in the Beyond as our physical body does in this world, made an indelible impression on me when I first read the article several years ago. Of course, the idea itself was not new to me, it is the central idea of *The Secret of the Golden Flower*, for example, but the penny at last dropped, so to speak, when I read this clear formulation of it in Wilhelm's article. It is not even an exclusively Eastern idea, the Western alchemists also often emphasize this quality of their lapis. Only to quote one example, the *Rosarium Philosophorum* says: "We have seen it with our own eyes and touched it with our hands." And, in his Eranos lecture, "On Zosimos," in 1937, Jung suggests that Christ was referring to the same thing when he said to Nicodemus: "We speak that we do know, and testify to that we have seen" (John 3:11).[11]

What subtle substance exists that is as tangible and visible as these testimonies suggest? All I can think of must be something similar to the ectoplasm that mediums produce in séances. Numberless scientifically controlled experiments with the weight of mediums during séances—to

---

[10]Wilhelm, "Death and Renewal in China."

[11]C. G. Jung, "The Visions of Zosimos," in *The Collected Works*, vol. 13 (Princeton, N. J.: Princeton University Press, 1967), pp. 57-108.

say nothing of the many photographs that have been taken–have proved that this ectoplasm has a physical weight and is sufficiently visible to register on a sensitive enough film. But the results of such séances are usually exceedingly primitive and unsatisfactory, and most parapsychological phenomena are particularly frequent in the neighborhood of adolescents who have not yet become conscious of the great change that is taking place in them.

In fact, altogether parapsychological phenomena seem often to be the pre-stage, as it were, of a creative effort. Jung used sometimes to say: "There were loud reports in the furniture in my room last night, so evidently I have to make another creative effort but I am not yet conscious of its content." And you will all remember the dramatic account he gives in *Memories* of the parapsychological phenomena that took place all over his house before he wrote "The Seven Sermons to the Dead."[12] The haunting ceased immediately when he took up his pen to write.

Altogether–although, of course, we are speaking of something which in itself is beyond our comprehension–parapsychological phenomena seem to point to a condition of the beginning, a condition in which the ectoplasm, so to speak, is still entirely autonomous. A creative effort, a becoming conscious, the "thoughts and works" mentioned by Wilhelm, seem to crystallize it, as it were, and thus to begin to form the "subtle body" which he speaks of here, a sort of mandalalike refuge of an enduring kind.

I admit that I thought concretely enough, when I first read of this formulation of Wilhelm's, to think that this subtle body must necessarily resemble the physical body in shape. Presumably it has this aspect. Jung's dream of the Yogin–to which we will return later–who had his features points in this direction.[13] And his experience in 1944 when he saw his doctor in his primal form telling him he must return to earth–he evidently recognized him at once–is also similar evidence.[14] To say nothing of the Zen masters who sometimes say to their pupils, "Show me your face before you were born." But obviously as this body is thought of as our refuge in the Beyond, it must belong to a realm where we are entirely dependent on symbols as the best possible expression for something that is essentially unknown. In *Memories,* Jung spoke of the

[12]Jung, *Memories,* p. 189ff.

[13]Ibid., p. 323.

[14]Ibid., p. 292.

yellow castle in the Chinese *Secret of the Golden Flower* as such a symbol and calls it directly "the germ of the immortal body."[15]

There is really a great deal of evidence to be found in modern dreams that the Western unconscious is just as concerned with our building "a subtle body of a spiritual nature" already in our lifetime as in China. I will just draw your attention to two examples. A woman–who was still under fifty–had a particularly clear dream in this respect. She was at the time much occupied with the problem of whether to buy a certain house. She was very anxious for some comment from the unconscious before making her decision irrevocable, but to her great disappointment, she had no dream. Then, just before she completed the purchase, she dreamed that, though the house in question was quite suitable as a garage for her body, it was of little importance. Another house was of vital importance, and she should give her whole attention to building it. Already in the dream she realized that this house was in the Beyond, for its site was quite close to the house of a great friend who had died two or three years before.

A few months before his death, Dr. Jung told us that he had had a dream that the "other Bollingen," was now complete. I must explain that he had had several dreams throughout the later years of the "other Bollingen," which was apparently built in stages similar to the stages in which he built his Tower on the upper lake of Zürich, as he describes in his *Memories*.[16] From how he had always spoken of the "other Bollingen," we had no doubt that it was built on the boundary of the two worlds or even quite in the Beyond. So the news from his dream that it was now completed made us very sad, as one could not doubt that he himself felt that he would move into it entirely before long.

Wilhelm points out that the physical body itself is quite willing to die when its time comes but that there is an inner aspect of the body that possesses consciousness and it is this aspect which is constantly imagining how death will be before it comes. It is this aspect that gives rise in many, if not most individuals to a profound desire for immortality, and which is constantly imagining how death itself will be. Wilhelm regards these fantasies as one of the strongest forces there is, that has created such buildings as the pyramids but also–ironically enough–killed millions of people in religious wars between people who held conflicting fantasies as to how it should be. The old philosopher, Dschuang Dzi, held that the psyche can be taken apart, as it were, and that conscious-

---

[15]Ibid., p. 197.

[16]Ibid., p. 223.

ness can learn to stand aside and watch the change in all things, an exercise that frees the ego from its body and immensely enlarges its range.

This taking apart of the psyche, and teaching the ego to stand aside and watch, seems to me very similar to what we do when we learn in analysis that the ego is not the master in its own house but only one of many inhabitants. Although we frequently try to manage the shadow, anima or animus, for instance, when we first learn how much they take upon themselves, it is really a good deal wiser and in the end more rewarding to stand aside and watch their behaviour till we know who or what they are. Moreover—as Jung was always emphasizing in analysis—the vital point is not what we are going to do about a thing, but whether we know it or not. Nothing could annoy him more than for us to ask: "What shall I do about it?" "Know it," he used to reply and sometimes remind us of *The Secret of the Golden Flower,* saying: "Indolence of which a man is conscious and indolence of which he is unconscious are a thousand miles apart."[17] If one can learn to stand aside and watch the "taken-apart psyche"—as Dschuang Dzi recommends here—we shall indeed see "the change in all things" for everything unconscious changes when it becomes conscious. This does indeed begin to free the ego from the body and to "immensely enlarge its range."

But this is not enough, as Wilhelm points out; the position must then be consolidated and that involves a separation from the corporeal altogether, and for that it is necessary to build up a new body for ego-consciousness. This body is made, as it were, of energy and can only be achieved by exercises in concentration and meditation to free these energies and to direct them to the support of the entelechy, that seed which is present from the beginning in latent form.

The seed that is present from the beginning but in latent form is, in our language, the Self. Jung has often compared it being there from the beginning with the lattice of a crystal which—though invisible—is present in the solution from the beginning. If, for a moment, we consider the making of this subtle body as if it were a crystal, the Chinese idea would roughly be, that the crystal itself could never form in the solution unless we spend the most profound meditation and concentration upon it which would enable it to become visible, hard and strong in the shape predestined from the beginning for that particular crystal.

Wilhelm carries this analysis of the seed further and points out how in every seed there is the image of a new plant or tree, but that—

[17]Wilhelm, *The Secret of the Golden Flower,* p. 91.

through concentration of the energy inwards—this image has become invisible, yet surrounded by a kind of substantial husk which must decay in order for the entelechy—the new image—to take on substance, develop, and become visible once more.

This image of the husk of a seed having to decay that the invisible entelechy may develop, again take on substance, and grow into the plant or tree is really the problem of rebirth, which—as Wilhelm points out—was regarded as so vitally important in the early centuries of Christianity but which no longer plays any role in the Church, at all events not in the Protestant Church. Yet, as Jung pointed out in his 1939 Eranos lecture, "Concerning Rebirth," all ideas of rebirth are founded on the fact that transformation of the psyche is a natural process.[18] He continues: "Nature herself demands a death and a rebirth. As the alchemist Democritus says: 'Nature rejoices in nature, nature subdues nature, nature rules over nature.' There are natural transformation processes which simply happen to us, whether we like it or not, and whether we know it or not."[19] It seems to me that the Confucians especially made a great effort to become conscious of the natural process of rebirth and to prevent it taking place unconsciously. That the latter can be disastrous beyond measure we saw in the last world war, for, as I am sure all of you remember, Jung pointed out repeatedly that the events in Germany were simply an individuation process taking place in the unconscious, with no one aware of it.

Jung spoke particularly plastically of the undeveloped seed idea in his 1932 seminar on Kundalini yoga. He pointed out that the fact of our still being in *Muladhara* shows that we are still just seeds of what we could become, less than embryos, only germs in the womb.[20] These germs are the sleeping gods, what we should call the Self, which lie invisible and latent in us all. Jung even says:

> What we take to be the culmination of a long history and long evolution would be really a nursery, and the great and important things are high above it and are still to come; exactly as the unconscious contents which we feel down below in our abdomen are still rising to the surface and becoming conscious so that we begin to have the conviction,

---

[18]C. G. Jung, "Concerning Rebirth," in *CW*, vol. 9i (Princeton, N.J.: Princeton University Press, 1959), pp. 113–150.

[19]Ibid., p. 130.

[20]J.W. Hauer, "Kundalini Yoga," Seminar at Psychological Club, Zürich, 1932, p. 154.

> this is definite, this is clear, this is really what we are after.[21]

Jung goes on to point out that while this is only a germ, it is apt just to disturb our functioning, but that—if we persevere in concentrating on it—it becomes an embryo and even—when it fully reaches consciousness—it becomes a full-grown tree. He points out that the whole purpose of the awakening of the Kundalini is to separate the gods from the world—where they have slept—so that they may become active, and with that we necessarily start a new order of things. He adds:

> From the standpoint of the gods, this world is less than child's play, it is a seed in the earth, a mere potentiality, our whole world of consciousness is only a seed of the future. But when you succeed in the awakening of Kundalini, so that she begins to move out of her mere potentiality, you necessarily start a world which is a world of eternity, totally different from our world.[22]

As we shall see, the goal of all that Wilhelm tells us in this paper is really exactly the same as Jung describes here, it is becoming conscious of the *world of eternity* but it adds the idea of forming a new body in which we can find a refuge in this world of eternity, just as the physical body is our home and refuge in this world.

We have learned so far that this subtle body is made of "thoughts and works" and above all of energy, which we must detach from the earthly things—that have been our main preoccupation—and give to supporting and furthering this entelechy, this seed of the eternal that is latent in us all. Only a movement of retreat with the utmost concentration, Wilhelm says, makes it possible for the new growth to take root, and Jung pointed out in his Kundalini seminar that when this seed begins to move in us, it has "the effect of an earthquake that naturally shakes us and can even shake our house down."[23] We obviously need strong roots in the "here and now" to stand this, and I think it is just here that the Chinese better consciousness of the earthly body stands them in good stead and has probably contributed a lot to their being more willing and able than we are "to form a conception of life after death or to create some image of it."[24]

---

[21]Ibid., p. 156.

[22]Ibid.

[23]Ibid., p. 158.

[24]Jung, *Memories*, p. 302.

The necessary concentration is expressed in China through many images. Only to mention one: a sage is depicted in deepest meditation in whose heart a small child is forming. This little child is nourished and cared for there until at last it is ready to float through the cranial cavity into the heights as the new divine birth. This, Wilhelm says, is an image that represents death already in life. It means emerging into another order of time, where we can see the whole of life as from another dimension and yet, at the same time, we remain energically connected with our present life in our present order of space and time. Wilhelm says that this meditation engenders a concentrated latent energy which gathers everything to one point because it frees itself from transitory time. It is clear that no ordinary intellectual thinking would be of the slightest use here, in fact, the only Western parallels that I know are the profound meditation of the mystic and the concentration on the unconscious that Jung learned and taught us in active imagination.

Wilhelm points out that this is a point on which all the Chinese religions agree: Confucianism as well as Taoism and Buddhism all hold that the most important task of a lifetime is to bring every physical and psychic disposition, that form the capital with which we are born, into harmony by assembling them all round a center which then shapes them into a whole. He points out that if this procedure succeeds, it represents the most unusually strong force. The danger in the East, which Wilhelm points out, of not being able to keep all these psychic components together and of getting possessed by a force that escapes and becomes autonomous, is exactly the same as so often threatens us. An autonomous complex, such as the animus or anima, can gain the upper hand and even land us in a condition that is worse than before we made the attempt to reach our unconscious. Jung often used to deplore this fact and say that if people were not going through with it, it was better that they should never begin.

Wilhelm points out that such incidents–which are depicted in numberless fairy tales–are only of secondary importance in China where the recognized goal in all three great religions is to *unite* the whole psyche round a center by constant meditation and concentration. They say, indeed, that deviations from this goal make it possible, for example, to talk to the ghosts of the deceased. Although, as Wilhelm tells us elsewhere, mediumistic séances are "widely prevalent" in China, and we also learn that they are not valued at all highly by the Chinese who are concerned with the goal which we are considering.[25] Jung also tells

---

[25]Wilhelm, *The Secret of the Golden Flower*, p. 3.

us that outpourings of the unconscious, such as we frequently reckon as works of genius, are also not highly valued in China. (I imagine he means such works as Nietzsche's *Thus Spake Zarathustra*, which has all the characteristics of having burst forth from the unconscious with little or no control being exercised by the conscious.) Such works are regarded in China as wasted energy, undeveloped births, which finally—because they are not subjected to conscious concentration, and thus related to the center—flicker out and disappear.

It seems to surprise Wilhelm very much that, as he expresses it, something lower, like ego-consciousness, should have to take the lead in the production of something so much higher than itself that it could even be called divine. Yet the Chinese take this fact very seriously and say that at first this higher being needs to be educated and formed by consciousness, for it is powerless to develop without. We are already used to this idea, for the alchemists also say that the god hidden in matter can only be liberated by the efforts of the alchemist himself. And it is an archetypal idea that quite frequently appears in the dreams of modern people. For example, Dr. Jung once told me that a woman patient of his had the following dream: there was a group of birds, all about the size of pigeons, and she had the task of teaching them to walk up and down stairs. To her great surprise, one of these birds was the Holy Ghost, who had to be taught the same thing, exactly like the other birds. Dr. Jung remarked that this only sounded extraordinary because of our Christian upbringing, it was really just a natural fact.

So the Chinese undertake the education, or one could perhaps rather say the liberation, of this seed that is innate in us all. This, as we have seen, largely consists of freeing the energy that is caught up with all our worldly concerns and surrounding the entelechy with it. Or, in other words, freeing our minds of the finite in order to concentrate on the infinite which—while we are still alive—accustoms us to the Beyond and its infinite, unlimited values, before the time comes for us to move over or, in other words, to die.

Jung speaks just as strongly in his *Memories* of the value of realizing the infinite. He even says: "The decisive question for man is: Is he related to something infinite or not? That is the telling question of his life." But he adds the warning:

> The feeling for the infinite, however, can be attained only if we are bounded to the utmost. The greatest limitation for man is the "Self." It is manifested in the experience: "I am only that"! Only consciousness of our narrow confinement in the Self forms the link to the limitlessness of the unconsciousness. In such awareness we experience ourselves concurrently as limited and eternal, as both the one and the

> other. In knowing ourselves to be unique in our personal combination—that is, ultimately limited—we possess also the capacity for becoming conscious of the infinite. But only then![26]

Here, I think, is the point above all where any imitation of the East can harm us. They are conscious of "their narrow confinement," but all too often we are not. And yet—as Jung makes so clear here—it is the *conditio sine qua non* of all realization of the Beyond. Therefore, we cannot, as the Chinese do, fix our whole attention and concentration on the infinite—we get terribly out of ourselves if we try—but we can approach the same result by the paradox: "I am only that" and yet I can participate and to some extent realize the infinite at one and the same time.

The Chinese point out—and this probably also holds good for us—that the best opportunity to realize the infinite is in sleep. The philosopher Dschuang Dzi says that "the spirit wanders in sleep, for in sleep it is in the liver." Wilhelm explains that he means that during sleep it is not in the brain, nor anywhere in consciousness, but in the vegetative system. Deep sleep, they think, is very nearly related to the condition in which we shall find ourselves after death. But here their view is again different from ours in that they regard dreams as "remnants of consciousness" and think that they should be educated not to disturb us. This, to them, is the same thing as educating ourselves for life after death, and they maintain that great sages no longer dream.

This is always a great difference between the East and our own point of view. They seem, for the most part, to be entirely blind to the value of dreams and to how much we can learn from them about the condition they wish to establish. We certainly do not think it would help to educate our dreams (!), in fact, we know we can do nothing of the sort without grave psychic loss. Dr. Jung dreamt up to just before his death and most particularly meaningful dreams. But that we are in the Beyond during sleep, almost entirely freed from the limitations of space and time, is certainly an idea that is founded on fact.

This is probably the reason why it is possible for us to "do our best to form a conception of life after death, or to create some image of it." Probably the Beyond is much less strange and far more familiar than we expect. I once heard of an English doctor whose experience during a bad illness brings us some confirmation of this. He was very near death, in fact, the people round him had even thought he was dead, but nevertheless he recovered entirely. Afterwards he remembered very vividly,

---

[26]Jung, *Memories*, p. 325.

that he had been in a place which was even more familiar to him than his own house and garden. But he had been astonished beyond measure to learn that this familiar place was death. Dr. Jung—when he heard of this—said that exactly agreed with his own impression; he thought we should find the Beyond extraordinarily familiar to us. He added, however: "But I don't think the ego will like the change, we must reckon a protest from it."

Wilhelm then goes into what he calls a third subject, which is not individual but collective in character. As this would be rather long and complicated to explain, I would like to remind you of the better known and similar idea of the individual and universal Atman. Using that language, it is only through the existence of the universal Atman that it is possible for the individual Atman to experience the post-mortal condition in a way that no longer arouses the slightest fear. Therefore, it is the task of life to prepare itself for death—not in the sense of chalking up a number of good deeds to our credit in order to insure our later entrance into heaven, but in the sense of creating a condition that represents a detachment from the finite in favor of the infinite. This they regard as a journey or journeys into the universe.

A short time before his death, Dr. Jung dreamt that he saw a green, scarablike beetle circumambulating his pocket knife, spinning a thread round and round it. Then it went on to spin a sail, and using the pocket knife as an anchor, it sailed off into space. The pocket knife was one Dr. Jung had had for years and used daily for many purposes, so, if we take it as representing the ego mind and will, we might venture the hypothesis that—even in death—the ego does not just disappear but is put to a completely new use, i.e., it is used as an anchor to the individual which would prevent the soul from disappearing into the impersonal unconscious.

Wilhelm goes on to explain that detachment from the finite—whether it is in actual death or death in life for rebirth—is a repetition of the great psychical revolution of birth, when heaven and earth step aside and change places for the human being. If we think of Dr. Jung's dream of the Yogin who had his face and who, he realized, was the one either meditating or dreaming his present life, we might say that, at birth, the great figure of the Yogin, representing heaven, steps aside, or falls asleep, and gives over the action for its lifetime to the ego, representing the earth.[27] And, as Dr. Jung realized in his dream, when the Yogin wakes up and takes over again, the ego will cease to function as

[27]Ibid., p. 323.

before, either through actual death or by the ego's death for rebirth. The death of the ego for rebirth is really exactly what Meister Eckhart constantly advises when he says, "Leave yourself." He even says:

> Remember, in this life no one ever left himself so much but he could find something more to leave. Very few can stand it who know what it really means. It is just a give and take, a mutual exchange: thou goest out of things so much and just so much, no more or less, does God go in: with all of his if thou dost go clean out of all thine. Try it, though it cost thy all. That way lies true peace and none elsewhere.[28]

In his own Western, medieval language, Meister Eckhart is advising the same thing here as the Chinese do when they say they should detach their whole attention and energy from the finite and give it to the infinite. Meister Eckhart sees it as giving up our own human way entirely, so that God may replace it by His divine will, whereas the Chinese sage sees it as giving up all interest in the world so that the divine entelechy, that is present in us all, may develop and grow into its own realm, the infinite.

That these efforts—difficult as they are—sometimes succeed in China is demonstrated by the fact that Wilhelm tells us the different ways in which the Taoists and Confucians live after it has succeeded. Both indeed now take eternal things much more seriously than temporal matters. It seems, however, that the Taoist develops a very ironical attitude to this life and is inclined to despise and laugh at the whole thing. But the Confucian, Wilhelm says, shows a "sovereign dignity" in his whole new attitude to this life. He descends from the high summits he has discovered to the place on earth where he belongs and most adequately fulfills every duty which pertains to that place. This is not, Wilhelm adds, because he feels any need to acquire merit by doing so, but because it is now the way which it suits him to live. He can give himself fully to this life now because he no longer has any need to go over into the Beyond. Finite and infinite, here and Beyond, are no longer in any way separated for him, they exist simultaneously and are both penetrated equally by the Tao, the meaning, in which he now lives and has his being.

At bottom the idea of the Confucian now living his life in Tao is exactly what Meister Eckhart also means when he says that, if we can only give up our own ego way entirely, God will replace it completely by

---

[28]P. deB. Evans, trans., *Meister Eckhart*, vol. 2 (London: John Watkins, reprinted 1952), p. 6.

His will. It is really only a difference in language, for in both cases we live by something that is equally at home in finite and infinite, to such an extent that the two are no longer separated by space or time. Or–to put it in our own more modern language–the ego abdicates in favor of the Self. But–and this is very important for us–we, like the Confucians, must then live our outer lives more and not less fully. Dr. Jung said in his seminar on Kundalini:

> You should leave some trace in this world which notifies you have been here, that something has happened. If nothing happens of this kind, you have not realized yourself, and the germ of life has fallen into a thick layer of air that kept it suspended, it never touched ground, so could never produce the plant.

And he adds later: "If you succeed in completing your entelechia, that shoot will come up from the ground, namely the possibility of detachment from this world."[29]

Only by detachment–that quality which Meister Eckhart values higher than any other–can we "form a conception of life after death or create some image of it."[30] But we can only afford this detachment by the utmost attachment to life and by a determination to live it as faithfully as possible, till we really come to the right time for, what the Chinese call, the greatest good fortune of all: namely finding our own specific death, which will crown and not tear apart our life.

---

[29]Hauer, p. 161.

[30]deB. Evans, *Meister Eckhart*, vol. 1, pp. 340ff.

Introduction to the Cat, Dog, and Horse Seminar

The Cat, Dog, and Horse Seminar was one series of the many lectures delivered by Barbara Hannah at the Psychological Club. This club was founded by Jung in 1916 because, as Miss Hannah explained, "people in analysis badly needed a place where they could find others with the same interests, exchange views, and find companionship."

Miss Hannah's lectures were carefully written, and her individualistic delivery style was characterized by much feeling and spontaneity. She laughed easily, often, and heartily. She paused often to invite questions or comments. In her later lecturing years, she lamented that class size did not permit opportunity for discussion, as in the past. The large class size was evidence of her popularity as a lecturer. She continued to lecture until she was eighty-five.

When criticized for quoting Jung so much, she mentioned that Jung had also criticized her for quoting him so much. Her reply to Jung was: "I can't help it; that is how it is. I have learned these things from you and I must acknowledge that. I don't know another way to do it honestly."

A student recalled that when Miss Hannah lectured, she would bring "half a library" with her. Those who heard her were impressed, not only with her knowledge, but with her unquestioning belief in the importance of the unconscious and in the immediate reality of the animus and anima.

A woman who heard her lecture for the first time said, "That was a profound experience; she helped me understand things in a different way." Another person said, after hearing her lecture, "She must have gone very deep into her own analysis to be able to talk like that."

Cat, Dog, and Horse Seminar: Lecture 1

April 26, 1954

Animals almost invariably represent instincts when we meet them in dreams and active imagination. Each animal represents a different instinct or, if you prefer it, another aspect of instinct. As we discuss our separate animals, particularly their mythology, we shall see how many-sided they are and that the meaning necessarily depends on context in the dream and the conscious situation of the dreamer. It is too cheap to hang a ticket around the neck of an animal and always take the cat, for instance, as a woman's catty feminine nature, or as the anima cat, or to mention witchcraft vaguely, as the cat is undoubtedly a witch animal, a stigma it shares, however, with a great many other small animals, such as hares, mice, rats, snakes, toads, spiders, ravens, crows, and so on. The cat does have a great deal to do with feminine nature, and the anima is very often a cat, but it has many other shades of meaning which appear in its actual characteristics, and still more in its mythology. One needs to know something at least about these before one can be at all sure what a cat is likely to represent in individual dreams and fantasies. Hanging a label about the animal's neck is really as bad as the labeling system of the Freudians, which we are always ready to criticize. An animal—and every animal is different—has at bottom something intensely mysterious which lies beyond our powers of comprehension. We can only attempt, by considering the animal itself as we know it and its mythology, to get some idea of the quality and meaning of its specific mysterium.

As a general rule there is, to me at least, something relaxing or reassuring in dreaming about an animal, though of course this again depends on the context, but one often gets the feeling of a return to nature and of being reunited to something very healing.

In an unpublished paper on the transcendent function, Jung says that to go back to nature in the primitive sense would be a mere regression, but to strive to reach it through psychological development is something quite different, for this time it means doing consciously what before we did unconsciously. Therefore, it is obvious that if we follow our animals back into nature, we must on no account lose our hard-won consciousness. If we can achieve this, however, we shall find it restful, for we shall be going with the stream instead of battling against it.

Except in very rational situations, we are able to do very little without the help of our instincts, and one of the most threatening symptoms of the present day is the extent to which many people are divorced from them. The primitive, as you know, can do hardly anything without a sort of *rite d'entrée*. As an example, Jung has sometimes told the story of one of his boys in Africa to whom he gave a letter with instructions to deliver it, but, as this proved useless, he went to the head boy who gave the messenger a long talk, impressing upon him his importance as a go-between between two great chiefs, with the result that the man started off to run the whole twenty miles without a stop.

As far as our superior functions are concerned, the efforts of many generations have detached a certain sum of energy which is under the control of the will, and there we are entirely dependent on the instincts. Further, we experience the same phenomenon the moment we touch our inferior function. For these reasons, I think we may find it very helpful to study the archetypal images of three animals that represent instincts which—like the animals themselves—are very close to us, perhaps the closest.

The Curatorium asked me to speak on this subject. As it is not a theme on which I have been working for years, like the ego and shadow, the animus, active imagination, or the Brontës, I felt a certain reluctance, but was struck by the fact that these were the three animals with which I have had most to do in my own life, though I should like to have had months, instead of a few weeks, in which to prepare the material.

One point about which we must be as clear as possible from the beginning is the difference between instinct and archetype. They could be called two aspects of the same thing, as they have a secret connection which can be exceedingly confusing. For the sake of clarity, therefore, I will read you Dr. Jung's definitions in "Instinct and the Unconscious" in *Contributions to Analytical Psychology:*[1] "Instincts are typical ways of action and reaction, and whenever it is a matter of uniformly and regularly repeated actions, we are witnessing instinct. It is quite indifferent whether there is an association with conscious motivation or not." "Archetypes are typical forms of apprehension; indeed, wherever we meet with uniformly and regularly recurring ways of apprehension they are referable as archetypes. It is also quite indifferent whether the mythological character is recognized or not." As an illustration, there is the

---

[1]CW 8, par. 273, 280.

famous story of Socrates' daemon which whispered to him to turn to the right, by which he escaped being trampled down by a herd of wild swine. We can call this archetypal, for he heard his daemon speaking, i.e., he apprehended it from within. But if he had acted blindly, turning into the other street with no idea why, it would have been blind instinct. Instinct is an automatic outer way of behaving, whereas archetype is a disposition for apprehending the inner meaning.

In the summer of 1931, in the first volume of the Visions, Jung says that animals represent the lower instinctive forces in man and gives, as one of his examples, the fact that a horse often knows the way when the rider feels completely lost. Later, in the same seminar, he gives a practical example of a woman who was working with him and who had very suicidal ideas. She had made up her mind to throw herself into the lake, but, on the way, saw in a shop a pair of shoes she liked and after buying them her wish to die had completely left her. Jung likens this to a camel which might have passed her in the desert and shown her the way she had completely lost. In fairy tales and myths the helpful animal often saves the hero by showing him something nearby and self-evident which he just had not seen; sometimes they do even more and bring the whole solution. In all natural situations, Jung says, the instincts are far better protection than all the intellectual wisdom in the world, though in most civilized situations we require the mind, and instinct would only lead us deeper into the soup. It is always a case of Scylla and Charybdis, for if we stay too long with our instincts, we might indulge in them and lose our consciousness entirely, and if we live entirely in the mind, we are lost in the natural situations of which our lives largely consist.

Jung often speaks of the piety of animals and of how much nearer they live to God's will–to their true nature–than we do. He frequently quotes the logion in the Oxyrhynchus Papyrus where Christ is asked what draws us to the Kingdom of Heaven and gives the answer, the fowls of the air, all the beasts upon and under the earth, and the fishes of the sea. In the Visions (vol. 1, p. 139) he says:

> That means the instincts; the blind instincts almost; the way of nature will bring you quite naturally to wherever you have to be. That is the idea of Tertullian, *anima naturaliter christiana,* meaning the soul is naturally Christian, in other words, a natural process leads on to the Christian formulation.

This, of course, applies to the people whose natural law coincides with Christianity. Jung adds later that if you follow the way of nature, you will quite naturally come to your own law.

> Then one comes to the question, what is the law of man? According to preconceived ideas he is all wrong, sinful, little better than an earthworm. But that is an absolutely wrong idea. Who has created the religions of the world? Man! If left to himself, he can naturally bring about his own salvation. Who has produced Christ? Who has produced Buddha? All that is the natural growth of man. Man has always produced symbols that redeemed him, so if we follow the laws that are in our own nature, they quite naturally will lead us to the right end. (Visions, vol. 1, p. 139)

He goes on to point out that that is just what active imagination can do for us. Our fantasies do not lead us straight to hell (unless we indulge in them and use active imagination in the wrong way) but, if we learn to trust our own experience, it will, according to the natural law, lead us to a state of completeness, to what we really are. I must emphasize that it is not a case of simply following the instinct but of seeing the meaning of it. In Visions, Jung says:

> The original unconscious primitive condition of man is a sort of rock that contains gold, and if you put that body through such a chemical–or, in this case, psychological–treatment, the rock will yield gold; that is an analogy for the so-called transformation of instincts. You simply separate certain instincts that were contained in the original unconscious, you lift them up into consciousness, and so you naturally change the original condition of the primitive man, he becomes conscious; consciousness is the gold that has been before contained in unconscious, but so distributed that it was invisible. There is a lot of gold in the unconscious of primitive man; his unconscious is different from ours, and it shows far more signs of vitality; our unconscious still occasionally behaves in the same way but only when we are unconscious as primitive man is continuously. Through the process of civilization you bring out slowly all the gold and other previous metals that were contained in the original unconscious; the philosopher's stone, the diamond, the gold, the *elixir vitae*, the fluid that makes you immortal, etc., all these are symbols for the various substances extracted from that rock of original unconsciousness. Through that process things surely change, but if you make a solution of the gold and pour it into the heap of ashes, in time it will form a rock as before. So if you allow your consciousness to be dissolved, you will create again the original unconsciousness, because everything is there. In this respect we have not transformed the instincts, we have only taken out of them something which they contained. For instinct is merely the unconscious mental functioning of man, in which there are the possibilities of extracting the gold of consciousness.

We see here the vital importance of keeping consciousness intact. Dr. Baynes once more or less expressed the same thing in the simile of a boat. At first, in natural consciousness you went blindly with the current till you hit a snag or came to grief in the rapids. Then, warned by the catastrophe, you learned to row against the stream and you usually went on doing that till you collapsed with exhaustion. And then only were you ready to learn both ways: i.e., to let your boat go with the stream and use your consciousness to steer.

Again, in Visions, Jung says:

> You see, in practical psychology, there is always the great and important question for the analyst whether a series of emotions is really correct, whether it is according to the instincts, that is. For if it is against the instincts, it is all morbid waste, but if the instincts are with it, you know it is all right, they belong, they are the right food, the correct magic procedure. And instinct is represented usually by an animal, a dog, a horse, an elephant; in this case, a buffalo is there as a sort of exponent indicating that it is correct, it is with the instinct.

Now in extracting the gold from these emotions that are with the instinct, the first thing to do is to make a difference between yourself and your own emotion. If you cannot do this, you are its prey, and you become a wild animal divorced from consciousness, simply dissolved in the unconscious; but when you are no longer identical, you begin to extract the gold from the heart of your instinct, you leave *Manipura* and enter *Anhata* where you catch your first glimpse of the *Purusha*. The Eastern point of view is much better based on the instincts than ours. We always think we can command our instincts whereas we really can do nothing of the kind. We can merely learn to accept them, and to disidentify with them and thus extract some of the gold of their archetypal meaning.

Before we turn to our actual animals, I should like to make an attempt to show how such images fit into our psyche and how we are to regard them psychologically. I would like to read you a few passages I have translated from Dr. Jung's last book, *Von den Wurzeln des Bewussteins*, in which "Geist der Psychologie" appears under the new title "Theoretische Ueberlegungen zum Wesen des Psychischen" (Theoretical Reflections Concerning the Essence of the Psychical). Dr. Jung says:[2]

---

[2]*CW* 8, par. 387.

> The light of consciousness has—as we know from direct experience—many grades of intensity and the ego complex many levels of emphasis. On the animal, or primitve level, there is a mere luminosity, which it is hardly possible to distinguish from the luminosity of dissociated fragments of the ego. On an infantile and primitive level, consciousness is not yet a unit, for it is *not* centered around a firmly established ego complex but flickers up here and there wherever it is aroused by outer or inner events, instincts, or emotions. On this level it still has an insular character, or that of an archipelago. Even on a higher level, or on the highest level, consciousness is still no fully integrated totality, but is rather capable of an indefinite extension. Flickering islands—if not whole continents—can still be added to a modern consciousness, a phenomenon which has become an everyday experience for the psychotherapist. Therefore, one would be wise to think of ego-consciousness as being surrounded by many small luminosities.

This already gives us a valuable hint as to how we can regard our instincts. Unless they are extraordinarily integrated, they are like dim luminosities, which surround the consciousness of our ego complex, luminosities that can guide us in places where our ego consciousness is not yet up to the situation.

Jung speaks of how Paracelsus regarded these luminosities, the *lumen naturae* as he and many of the other alchemists call them. Jung says:[3]

> In respect of our hypothesis of multiple phenomena of consciousness, it seems to me above all important that with Paracelsus the characteristic alchemistic vision—of gleaming sparks in the dark secret substance—should be changed into the spectacle of an *inner firmament and its stars*. Paracelsus regards the dark psyche as the starry nocturnal sky, whose planets and constellations represent the archetypes in their whole luminosity and numinosity. The starry sky is actually the open book of cosmic projection, the mirror image of mythology, i.e., of the archetypes. From this point of view, astrology and alchemy, those two antique representations of the psychology of the unconscious, shake hands.

Paracelsus was directly influenced by Agrippa von Nettesheim, who also assumes a "luminosity of *sensus naturae*." (Literally, "sense of nature." Dr. von Franz says it actually means being instinctively or intuitively linked with the whole surrounding cosmic nature.) It is from this

---

[3]*CW* 8, par. 392.

that clairvoyant or prophetic luminosities descend on four-footed animals, birds, or other living creatures and enable them to foresee future events. Agrippa quotes the *sensus naturae* from William of Paris (Guilielmus Partisiensis–first half of the thirteenth century). He wrote many works which influenced Albertus Magnus. William of Paris assumes that the *sensus naturae* has a higher sense than the usual human form of perception, and he particularly emphasizes that animals also possess it. The teaching of the *sensus naturae* developed from the earlier idea of a world soul which permeated everything. The world soul represented a natural force that was held responsible for all the phenomena of life and the psyche.

In Jung's later paper on synchronicity, he speaks of an "absolute knowledge" which is really a later formulation of this same phenomenon.

I should like particularly to emphasize Paracelsus's idea of the dark psyche as an inner firmament. For one could really regard the archetypal images of the cat, dog, and horse as stars in such an inner firmament and say that we intend to study these particular stars through the telescope as well as we can. We shall indeed find that all our three animals are constantly connected with the moon and the sun. Moreover they appear in the naming of the actual stars. There are the constellations Canis Major (great dog) and Canis Minor (little dog) known better for their brightest star, Sirius, which name is connected with the Greek adjectives meaning "scorching"; hence the "dog days" in August. The horse also appears in the heavens as Pegasus. I do not think there is an actual cat star–even my usual encyclopedia, Dr. von Franz, did not know one–but the cat's first cousin, Leo (the lion) appears as the fifth sign of the zodiac, thus also connected with August.

The book *Geist der Psychologie* is just coming out in English and when it does, I should like to recommend Chapter Seven on the pattern of behavior and archetype. There is another passage of which I would like to remind you, as it will help us to distinguish between animals and instincts, as patterns of behavior and as archetypal images, i.e., as their meaning. I refer to the passage we discussed in connection with Tobit, where Jung speaks of a kind of scale of consciousness. He says:[4]

> The psychic processes behave rather like a scale along which consciousness glides. Sometimes it finds itself in the neighbourhood of the instinctive processes and comes under their influence, sometimes it approaches the other end,

---

[4]*CW* 8, par. 408–409.

> where the spirit predominates and even assimilates the opposing instinctive processes. These opposite positions—both of which produce illusions—are by no means abnormal phenomena; on the contrary, they each represent a one-sidedness that is typical of the modern normal man. This one-sidedness, of course, does not only manifest in the two opposites, spirit-instinct, but in many other forms that I have depicted to some extent in *Psychological Types*. This "gliding consciousness" is very characteristic of the human being of today. The one-sidedness which it causes can only be overcome by realization of the shadow.

We will not go into this aspect of the realization of the shadow, for it belongs in another course, beyond saying that for many people today the shadow is very much connected with the instincts. Or perhaps I should say that it is difficult to get a clear view of the instincts because of their contamination with the unrealized shadow. We also, of course, often meet the opposite phenomenon, people who are on very good terms with their instincts and whose shadow is actually intellectual, the enemy of their instinctive behavior, and which will constantly try to confuse them in this respect and twist or destroy their natural reaction.

Jung says about this scale later:[5]

> Through active imagination one is put in a position where one can discover the archetype, and indeed not just by sinking into the instinctive realm, which would lead only to an unconsciousness which is incapable of differentiation or—worse still—to an intellectual substitute for instinct. Speaking in terms of the visible spectrum, this would mean that the *image* of the instinct is not to be found at the red, but at the violet end of the color scale. The dynamic instinct lies, so to speak, in the infrared, whereas the image is to be found in the ultraviolet.

Later he adds:[6]

> The realization and the assimilation of the instinct never takes place at the red end—that is, not by sinking into the instinctive realm—but by assimilating the image, which also means and evokes the instinct but in a totally different form to that which we meet on the biological level.

---

[5]*CW* 8, par. 414.

[6]Ibid.

Please do not take me too literally when I suggest that we shall meet the real animal—and the blind instinct it represents as such in us—at the infrared end of this scale and its archetypal image at the ultraviolet, but I think it would be well to keep this in mind, for it may help us a good deal in our difficult theme.

When in great uncertainty as to how to arrange these lectures, it was the cats that came to my rescue in the following dream:

> *I dreamed I walked down a long garden path and went into a large room where I had not been for years. There I found eight cats and was terrified that they had been neglected, but I found a young man was with them and that they were all right and well liked. Four walked in formation and four remained behind.*

Now my idea in the lectures is to follow the pattern of the dream something in the way of the cross hairs of a telescope. Dr. Jung at Ascona one year told some of us that we were inclined to be too critical of lectures because we looked at them from our own point of view, instead of taking the trouble to find out the point of view of the lecturer, as he expressed it, the cross hairs that he was using in his telescope. Of course, these cross hairs are a human device for measuring the scale or for limiting the sky, and you do not find them in the material itself.

The cross hairs I propose using are the four aspects of the concrete animal in the outer world, more or less corresponding to the instincts themselves. I shall amplify these four aspects by corresponding mythological material and attempt thus to find their archetypal meaning. With the much greater, overabundant material which we have for dog and horse, it would be more difficult to keep to the pattern, but for the cat it is easier. The fact that my dream, however, picked on a double quaternity is certainly no accident, for each of the animal instincts is a totality in itself, though it is at the same time only a part of the whole. There would be no Sahara without the individual grain of sand, as Jung says. The microcosm is just a small image of the great macrocosm.

Although on dogs we have an excellent book, *Hundesstammvater und Kerberos* by Freda Kretschmar, there is less material on the cat. For instance, it is never mentioned in the Bible and practically not in such books as Keller's *Animals of Classical Antiquity,* and hardly ever in the seminars or books of Dr. Jung.

I have given the dog the middle place because he is often nearly related to the cat in mythology, and also at times to the horse, whereas so far I have found little or no relationship between horse and cat. Also in outer stories, I know far more of friendships between cats and dogs, in spite of their traditional enmity, and of dogs and horses than between cats and horses, though I have heard of such stories. For instance, there is the one of the racehorse who, when in order to run in a race had to be separated from his friend, a cat, moped so terribly that the cat had to be sent for, but in my experience cat-and-horse stories are rare.

The cat is the least domesticated of our household animals. According to Brehm, it has been a domestic animal for about 4,000 years, whereas there were domesticated dogs in the Stone Age, therefore perhaps time plays a role in the cat's domesticity, but it is more probable that it is its essential character. Unlike the dog, it is an evasive animal and does not submit completely and live with us entirely. It is also more bound to the place than to the person. Professor Hediger, in a recent lecture at the institute, spoke of the, so to speak, elastic band which held the animal to its territory, and of the difficulties animals experience when they go beyond their usual radius. The cat is the only one of the domesticated animals which keeps its elastic band firmly attached to its home. Bombed-out cats in England were a great problem, for though their home might be in ruins, it was difficult to get them away from the place, so that it was quite a problem to feed and care for them. Their ability to find their way home over long distances is proverbial.

The dog, through domestication and his affectionate and loyal nature, has, to a great extent, transferred his elastic band to his master. There are exceptions, but most dogs will move quite happily with the people they love.

Horses are quite as attached to their stables as a cat to its home, but they settle down in a new stable very easily.

These are signs of long domestication, for it is much more difficult to move wild animals. Professor Hediger spoke of the difficulties connected with new arrivals at the zoo. People were apt to think that the animal would be so pleased to get loose, but where they had been transported in a cage, Professor Hediger made it a practice to let them, where possible, take their time in leaving this and moving into their permanent quarters, in some cases leaving the cage which had been their temporary home and to which they had become accustomed, inside the new quarters.

In one of the few mentions of cats in the Visions seminars, Dr. Jung remarks that cats—as the least domesticated of the domestic animals—resemble woman in this respect (Visions, vol. 2, p. 273). A dog is much more domesticated than a cat, just as man is more domestic than woman. This association of dogs with men and cats with women is practically universal.

We must first make a few general remarks about the cat as an actual animal.

THE CAT

The *Felidae*, or cat tribe, is a large family of which the domestic cat is only one branch. Brehm's *Thierleben* mentions lions, tigers, pumas, leopards, panthers, snow leopards, jaguars, and yet more as members of the true cat family. It may be wondered why I use an old-fashioned book like Brehm's when there are many more up-to-date books on the subject. No doubt if we were going to study animals purely from the biological or anatomical side, the newer books would be far better, for there would be a lot of new and valuable discoveries, but our purpose is to discover what animals mean to us psychologically, how they affect us, how we are to estimate a dog, cat, or horse when we meet them in dreams or active imagination and for this purpose Brehm remains *the* textbook par excellence, for he has no modern one-sided attitude but portrays a great deal of what man projects onto animals and that is just what we need to know. One could say that he describes animals not in modern scientific concepts, but in almost anthropomorphic terms. He says, for instance, that certain animals are tricky, fierce, ill-tempered, humorous, or the reverse, and so on, which is, of course, an application of human terms onto an animal that is really simply itself. A tiger is fierce or cruel when we look at it from our point of view, but from its own, it is simply obeying the law of self-preservation. When it sees a weaker animal, it sees a providential meal and to fail to add this tidbit to its larder would be to betray the law of self-preservation. It knows nothing of chivalry, protecting the weak and all that, so what meaning could the words *fierce* or *cruel* have from its point of view? But these words convey something of its nature to us, for they describe how we experience a tiger. We do not even pretend in these lectures to study animals just as they are. Therefore, the animal's anatomy and so on are only of secondary importance to us. These must, of course, be realized correctly; any illusions or delusions would be fatal. For instance, it matters in a dream whether an animal belongs to a warm- or cold-blooded species, whether it has a cerebrospinal system, what its biological functioning is, and so on; but it is much more important for us to realize the impressions each animal makes on man.

According to the *Encyclopedia Britannica*, the domestic cat is mainly descended from the Egyptian cat where North African wild cats were domesticated from very ancient days; according to Brehm, already about 2000 B.C. A late nineteenth-century naturalist, Dr. Nehring of Berlin, came to the conclusion that our domestic cat has a dual origin: Egyptian and Southeast Asian, i.e., from a Chinese, originally wild, cat which was domesticated. Most authorities, including Brehm, seem to take Egypt as their most likely origin and admit to possible crossing with

European wild cats, but mainly on account of the color of the pads of the paws. It seems to be most unlikely that our cats, with the possible exception of those with short, bushy tails, descend in any marked degree from tamed European wild cats. Therefore, for the most part, they are not indigenous to our soil. This Egyptian origin applies to the shorthaired breeds, especially the common tabby. Long-haired Persian or Angora cats, according to the *Encyclopedia Britannica,* come from the "manul" cat of the deserts of central Asia. Siamese cats do not seem certainly to originate in Siam.

MATERNAL AND FALSE NATURE

The female cat is a highly maternal animal. The cat seeks a hidden place for her kittens, largely because the tomcat, their father, would eat them if he found them. The cat mother is so maternal that she not only looks after her own family in a most exemplary and tender—but also, as they get older, in a highly educational—manner, but there are well-authenticated examples of mother cats who fed and brought up puppies, fox cubs, baby rabbits, hares, squirrels, rats, and even mice (Brehm and his small son made such experiments with their cats and confirmed this).

Brehm, who seems if anything a little prejudiced in favor of the cat, denies that they are false or vengeful, and says that everything depends on how they are treated and, though he emphasizes their attachment to the house, assures us that they can be almost as much attached to people. Many cat lovers tell us the same, and I have also met cats which seemed almost more attached to people than places. No doubt exceptional cats are capable of further domestication, but on the whole they remain amazingly independent and also the cruel and crafty hunter who will play with his living prey before eating it. They are, after all, a small edition of big, fierce beasts of prey, and if one loves a cat, one must love it as is and not try to de-cat it. In that respect they can teach us a lot in our relations to other human beings. It is also a fact which Brehm ignores that the cat is almost universally associated with magic and witches. The hook for this projection onto cats is probably the way that they, like serpents, with whom they have other similarities, can cast a sort of spell on their prey; a bird, for instance, is sometimes totally unable to fly away if it is caught in the spell of a cat's eyes.

Cats are, of course, immensely useful in ridding us of mice. Brehm tells us that Lehm made careful experiments and came to the conclusion that when mice were plentiful, every adult cat ate twenty mice a day on an average, i.e., 7,330 mice a year. The majority of cats also rid us of rats, though this requires more courage than every cat has. Cats go wild, as you know, very much more easily than dogs and really take to the woods and become poachers of every kind of game that is not too large for them. In contradistinction to dogs, a cat can support itself at large for years. On the other hand, a cat is one of the most cozy and relaxed animals that exist. They are just cozy when it suits them, however, for they are undoubtedly the most independent of all our domesticated animals. Kipling's immortal title of the cat that walked by herself is eternally true of even the most domesticated cat. We human beings easily regard them as false, for they change mood in what is to us an inexplicable way.

We might now attempt the cross hairs in our telescope as far as the actual cat, or our blind instinct that appears as a cat, is concerned.

I must emphasize once again, however, that the qualities, mainly taken from Brehm, I have attributed to cats in the following schema are already to a great extent human projections. A cat is just a cat, a just-so story, that follows its nature all of a piece. Whether it plays, hunts, sleeps, miaows, or purrs, it does so completely with the whole cat. The qualities which we attribute to it are human impressions, even in this first series referring to actual cats.

The examples in the second series – mainly from mythology – are, of course, still more human projections, just as mythology and astrology always are.

Naturally the cat provides us with hooks – they fit into its nature. As mentioned before, the fact that they are human projections is very helpful in finding out what they mean *to us* when we dream of them or have to analyze them in a patient's dream. Therefore, when we have established the main qualities of concrete cats – as we see them – we will go on to their mythology and then fit these aspects as well as we can into our scheme and finally try to see the psychological meaning of our examples and thus get an idea of what the cat may represent in unconscious material.

Clearly we cannot separate all these headings at all sharply. For instance, the mother cat can be just as, if not more, fierce and cruel than the hunter, and the cat that "walks by itself" and is intensely independent will also hunt when occasion arises.

Cat, Dog, and Horse Seminar: Lecture 2

May 3, 1954

We must first turn to Egypt, probably the original home of cats, for mythological material where aspects can be found which fit into all our four categories.

According to Bonnet in *Reallexikon der Aegyptischen Religionsgeshichte*, the cat cult in early times was more or less confined to the region of Bubastis (the delta of the Nile), which was the center of the worship of Bastet, the cat goddess. Bonnet says that in ancient times the cat was worshipped only at Bubastis. It was, however, worshipped sporadically in other places, but more anonymously, being referred to by such terms as "the beautiful one." Bonnet states that such small groups liked to get their nameless cats into the neighborhood of the great goddess. Bast, or Bastet, is referred to by the *Encyclopedia Britannica* as Ubast. In Egypt the cat goddess, Bastet, is very much mixed up with Sachmet, or Sechmet, the lion-goddess, and with the goddess Tefnut, who is also a lioness. In fact, even the famous Hathor, the heavenly cow, sometimes appears as a cat. Bastet and Sechmet are so much together that it is sometimes impossible to keep them apart.

Bastet is usually depicted with a human body and a cat's head. Tefnut is the sister-wife of Shu. These last two were originally worshipped as a pair of lions. Like Tefnut, Bastet was the daughter of Atun, the original creator god who appears in the pyramid texts as the chthonic original god. He is said to have impregnated himself and produced the first pair of gods – Shu and Tefnut – by spitting them out of his mouth. Dr. Jacobsohn mentioned this in a recent lecture and said there were other versions of how he produced them. As you know, Egyptian gods melt into each other and reappear in a confusing way amazingly like the way our own figures of the unconscious behave. When I had flu, I took notes which afterwards gave me the impression of having been deep into the unconscious and active imagination. There is nothing more like the unconscious, as we express it, than the Egyptian gods. We saw this in the lecture on active imagination and the world-weary man. Atun became Re, or Ra-Atun, that is, he became one with Ra, the sun god. In the German, he is spoken of as Re, but in

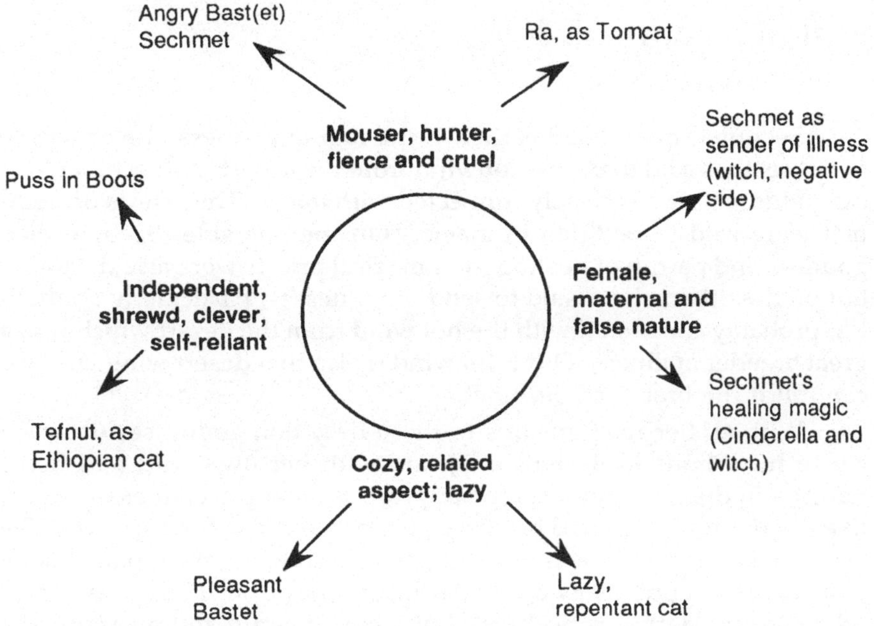

Figure 1. Aspects of the Cat

The Book of the Dead as Ra. Tefnut and Bastet appear later as daughters of Ra. In this role they usually appear as his moon (left) eye or, more rarely, as his sun eye, the right eye. In connection with Bastet, as the moon eye of the sun god, I should mention that according to Plutarch, the cat was directly connected with the moon. It is true that all these goddesses are found more often as the moon than as the sun, though Bonnet assures us that the cat itself is more a sun than a moon animal in Egypt and points out that a great many cat images have a scarab, a sun symbol, on their heads or breast. In the sun eye they are again contaminated with the serpent Uto and the culture goddess Mut. This is not surprising as cat and serpent have a good many common qualities. They have the same power of casting a spell on their prey and the same, to us, extraordinary unpredictable behavior. In later pictures of the sun god we find the bird who can also appear as a god. In such pictures the breast and head of a falcon usually grows out of the body of a cat, the reverse of the usual form of the cat head and the human body.

RAGE AND EMOTION

Sechmet, mentioned earlier, is the raging goddess of war whose fiery breath is said to be the hot wind from the desert. As Sechmet, our cat goddess Bastet is closely connected with magic. The priests of Sechmet were said to be "rich in magic." On the one side, Sechmet is a goddess and patron of healing–her magical priests were also doctors–but on the other, she is said to send out illnesses, particularly epidemics, probably connected with the hot wind from the desert which was a great breeder of illness. Our föhn wind is also that desert wind, and we can call it the breath of Sechmet.

With all her relationships to these fiery lion goddesses (it was a sin to hunt lions in Bastet's day) and with her own wild and fierce nature–in the pyramid texts she appears as an angry goddess–Bastet, like the domestic cat, had her very pleasant and comfortable side. The goddess Hathor, who was worshipped as a cow, the most placid of all animals, also appears as a cat. An inscription from Philae says that, when angry, Hathor is Sechmet, but when cheerful and pleasant, she is Bastet. Heroditus's description of the ecstatic Dionysian (in the sense of the adjective) festivals in Bubastis fit in here, where there was wine, dancing, music, and every kind of cheerful orgy. In Bubastis, huge cat cemeteries were found with mummified cats and many bronze representations of cats. In the pyramid texts, quoted by Dr. Jacobsohn a few years ago, prayers or charms for healing are seen to have been made almost as often for cats as for human beings. They were practically household gods. Dr. von Franz's sister, who was recently in India, said that it was tremendously striking to come from there, where cats were few and very wild, to Egypt where there are great quantities of beautifully kept domestic cats. It was a great sin in ancient Egypt to hit a cat and to kill one was terrible, but this is not confined to Egypt. Gubernatis, in *Zoological Mythology*, tells us that the cat is sacred to St. Martha in Sicily and is respected for her sake and that anyone who kills a cat is unhappy for seven years, like our mirror superstition. There is a well-known and very charming legend where Tefnut went off on her own to a distance as the Ethiopian cat and settled down in Nubis. Ra was very angry about this, so she used to sit on his forehead and spit at all his enemies, so he sent Thoth to fetch her back. In "La Religion des Egyptiens" by Adolphe Erman, there is a picture of her giving her paw to Thoth when she is going to let him take her back again.

In *The Book of the Dead*, it is reported that the sun god, Ra, himself fought as a tomcat against the Apophis serpent in Heliopolis.[1] A vignette shows him as a tomcat cutting off the head of the serpent. Bonnet thinks the cat was only the assistant of Ra in this battle, but nevertheless, "Great Tom Cat" is one of the names by which Ra is addressed. According to Bonnet, this battle may have been one of the causes of the cat becoming sacred in Egypt.

As a striking example of the cat's witchlike nature, under a positive aspect, I must mention the fact that in the Irish version of the Cinderella story the fairy godmother is replaced by a cat called Moerin. The witch, using destructive magic, would be the opposite of Moerin. The two aspects are very good examples of black and white magic.

We shall only be able to interpret the main theme of our stories just to get an idea of how the luminosity of the cat can help us when it appears in our dreams. To save time, we must keep to the role of the cat as much as possible and leave aside other motifs such as the Apophis serpent and Ra in the tomcat story. You probably know that the Apophis serpent is forever trying to destroy the sun boat of Ra when he is trying to get through the underworld, i.e., to destroy consciousness.

Beginning with Bastet in her wild and raging aspect—her Sechmet aspect—what do you think the image of such a cat might mean in a modern dream? It would be the raging, emotional side, probably very neglected feminine emotions or—in a man—a neglected anima who was just raging all over the place, a state of possession. The kind of day when the whole office says: "Look out, the boss is in a bad mood. Don't provoke him." Then the boss's anima is in her Sechmet aspect. Or, to take the case of a woman, a mistress who wakes up in a bad mood and takes it out on the cook, who in turn vents it on the kitchen maid, who takes it out on the cat! Quite right, in a way, since the cat was at the bottom of it. Only it is awful to project it onto the actual cat.

An Englishman with a very pronounced cat anima used to wake up in the night in such a mood, after having gone to bed feeling quite pleasant, and then everything went wrong. It usually began by his being furious with someone, and then he tormented himself with negative thoughts of every friend and everything in his life, the sort of mood in which one thinks of the atom bomb, and when nothing is of any use anyway. Once he dreamt, when he went to sleep after such a mood, that he was an adolescent boy and was tying a tin can onto the tail of a cat. Evidently the trouble began with his provoking or even torturing his anima cat, and she responded with a Sechmet mood of utterly negative

---

[1]Chapter 17, p. 103, of Budge's edition.

and destructive character. It is a case of the chicken and the egg. It is a fact that cats are very often tortured, much more often than dogs. This is presumably due to their independence and independent nature. They come in and eat, and then they go off, they do not make concessions, as dogs do. As to torturing, there was an interesting story in the paper the other day. Professor Hediger, now the Director of the Zürich Zoological Gardens, was trying an experiment with Rhesus monkeys, which have a most extraordinary social order. There is a head monkey who has a big harem, with first and second wives, and so on, down to the miserable no-class wives. He put in a young monkey, thinking he was too young to provoke the head monkey, but the least-important wife treated him so badly that he took to the water to get away from her. Hediger thought he would have to take him out when one of the head wives took him and made him delouse her and she deloused him, and then he was under her protection. The poor "bottom" wife had been so sat upon that as soon as this defenseless creature came, she could not resist the opportunity to torment him. The bother with the cat is that it usually wants the penny and the cake; it wants to eat our food, etc., but does not want to make any concessions. If you analyze such a mood with a man or a woman, you will usually find this psychology. The anima very often wants something very badly, but does not want to pay for it. It is the same with women when they get into these irrational angry moods. Such an angry mood can be symbolized by a fierce bull, but such anger is more aggressive, it has a purpose. In such a mood, a man might shoot his mistress, it has action, whereas the Bastet mood has not much action. In Sechmet moods, the man or woman will become more infantile. The Sechmet mood very often starts with being jealous and offended. A man is apt to become sentimental and to complain needlessly. An angry cat mood can be very sulky and resentful, there is no surrender in a cat, which can be very provoking. Angry cat moods provoke everybody around. I believe that the theory of the "jealous cat" is mainly a projection; dogs are much more jealous, but jealousy is often the cause of a Bastet mood. A man with a cat anima, or a woman with a catty nature like Bastet herself, can be very cozy and comfortable when the cat nature feels that way. Such a man, also, can purr around you and be quite delightful, but you never know when his claws are coming out.

In a story of Sechmet we get a hint of how such emotions can be used. The lord of heaven in the legend wished to send Sechmet out to destroy sinful man—not at all pleasant from man's point of view but, to the lord of heaven, quite practical because he can use the wild, emotional aspect for a definite purpose. This is also connected with the Sechmet magical aspect. In the Ra as tomcat story, there is a much more positive and differentiated aspect. When Sechmet is sent out, she can do anything she likes. Ra deliberately uses Sechmet for a definite purpose. He did not kill the Apophis serpent in his usual form as a sun god because he had to descend into the dark of the underworld where the sun has no place. But cats can see in the dark, so he made use of this instinct—the form of absolute knowledge expressed in the vehicle of the cat—to approach the serpent. A modern dream shows the two opposites which fought like Ahriman and Ormuzd. They were equal in strength for a long time, and the dreamer became afraid that the light figure would be defeated, when a small wraithlike fragment detached itself from the dark figure and went over to the light which then prevailed. There is the same motif in *Wuthering Heights*. The first Catherine was far too high, she did not take the mean cat qualities which were left to Isabella. The second Catherine behaved in a far more catty manner and at last was able to prevail against the negative animus of Heathcliff.

As to the common qualities of cat and serpent, both strike with the same lightning speed and can use surprise tactics unpredictably, so both are worthy foes and one sees why Ra chose to be a tomcat for this battle. Moreover, though the cat is a warm-blooded animal, it has some of the coldness of the serpent. Both are witches' animals and both are used in magic, but that is a stigma which they share with a great many other small animals, such as hares, birds, and so on. The important point is the nonidentification with the emotion and being able to differentiate from the mood and using it for a purpose. In a seminar here, someone once remarked that after all there were occasions when it is not a good plan to be too cool, that sometimes a certain emotion is needed, to which Jung agreed, but added that one should never use emotion unless you could just as well not use it, otherwise you would be possessed by it. If you felt that you would not be able to get through to a person without getting angry, as long as you feel a longing to let the anger loose, then don't; but when at last you can detach yourself and not be identical with it, and can say, "Ah, yes, that might be a way to get at that person," then you can. The one is an image of being possessed by emotion and the other of using it. There are situations where we cannot do anything with our consciousness. It is almost like the image of the Apophis serpent. If Ra had gone down as the sun, he would not have got anywhere near the serpent. To give an example: a girl I knew used to get on extremely badly with her mother and used to destroy herself by fighting, and the more she struggled, the more her rages and negative side got her. At last she thought she must find a way out, and then her hitherto useless anger became the incentive, and it stimulated her inventiveness till she actually found the solution. That is Ra fighting as a cat against the Apophis serpent, in contradistinction to the person caught in furious cat emotion and just letting it rip, when, of course, it works destructively, or at least extremely uncomfortably.

Remember that the lord of heaven sent out Sechmet to destroy mankind, and presumably Sechmet as the origin of illness belongs in the same connection. Here we enter the realm of witchcraft into which I do not want to go deeply. But there are many primitive stories of the witch doctor sending out the icicle or the bolt to hurt his enemies and afterwards having to be very careful because the bolt always comes back. A witch doctor would put his coat in the field so that the angry bolt should return to it instead of to him. Then he would rub it until it was quite tired and could put it in his pocket. The bad mood of the boss, or the cook, usually has no direction, so works more like a bad smell, making everyone miserable, or at least uncomfortable, to say nothing of the frightful waste of energy. A purpose always implies a certain detachment and this can be used positively as in the story of Ra or negatively as when Sechmet was sent out to destroy mankind. In nature, destruction and new growth are absolute opposites, but the one is necessary to make room for the other. If a tree did not become old and fall, there would be no place for the young tree. We enter here on a terribly difficult problem. You may all be angry with me when I say that sentimentality is partly responsible for the situation today. Before the first war, we were getting more and more sentimental. By helping to keep everything alive, we got too sentimental and destructive, and these dreadful wars broke out of us; when the one opposite is too much up, the other has to force its way through. Therefore we cannot avoid the fact that the destructive nature of the cat, which we cannot avoid, does show us that we have a hook for destruction in this instinct. Jung once said that it was no use to shut our eyes to the fact that if he is sitting in a chair, someone else cannot sit in it. To some extent we must push out other people to live, and we shall do it far better if we do it consciously and know what we are doing. Dr. von Franz in one of her lectures talks of the life of St. Niklaus von der Flue. Previously she herself had no idea of the enormous amount of worldly wisdom shown in it. It is a fact that he was a saint who did not eat for long periods, he was sustained in some way. The bishop, however, forced him to eat some bread, though St. Niklaus begged not to have to do it, saying it would make him ill, but he had to give in and became very ill, whereupon the Church agreed that his fasting was a fact. On being asked by a worldly troublemaker whether it was true that he did not eat, he was too clever to say "Yes," he merely replied, "God knows if it is true." Such an answer needed enormous detachment because one wants most dreadfully to justify oneself, but that is the evasiveness which is one of the most leading characteristics of the instinct of the cat. The dog is what he is, but the cat is more cunning.

In witchcraft every bolt returns to us. In a discussion on active imagination, Dr. Jung said that magic was really only in its right place when used subjectively on oneself – to destroy the vermin in ourselves. In active imagination there is a place where you can use fantasy in a very dangerous way, or it uses you as intrigues and plots and negative criticisms, etc., or you can use it positively in order to come to terms with your own unconscious. Or course, one has to use it as Niklaus von der Flue did, but we have to be dreadfully careful. One could say that the disease is the intrigue and the plot, and through accepting the fantasy one can do something about it. The unconscious can cause a neurosis and also heal it. Apollo could send the pest and could heal it, as could other gods, and Sechmet does the same. It is a complete paradox, but it accords with modern medical practice where the patient is inoculated with the disease itself. Who could know better how to heal than the originator? Quite obviously the one who sends the disease is *the* one who can heal it. Thus we have the cat as Cinderella's fairy godmother and the witch's cat, or the positive and negative aspect, the spinner of plots and intrigues and the highly positive subjective use.

COZINESS AND LAZINESS

When we come to the lazy side of the cat, the negative aspect of the cosy and comfortable side, one can turn to Tefnut, the Ethiopian cat who cut her duties; one could say that she was the initiator of the strike. To leave her owner, the ruler of heaven and the sun god, and go off on her own as she did was really the climax of independence.

On this aspect we find some good material in Gubernatis, *Zoological Mythology*.[2] In the "Pancatantram," the old Indian epic text, comparable to the *Iliad* and *The Odyssey* in Greece, there is a story of the cat "Butter Ears" or "White Ears" (the luminosity) who feigns repentance of all his crimes, so they think he must be wonderful and he is made a judge. Actually, in our own idiom, he has decided to let his head save his heels. As the repentant cat, he is asked to judge in a dispute between a hare and a sparrow. He pretends to be deaf and asks both to come a little closer and confide their troubles in his ears, whereupon he eats both – reconciliation takes place in his stomach and not quite in the way they had hoped.

---

[2]Vol. II, p. 42ff.

The cat is very shrewd and extremely false, but the decisive element is laziness here, since he gets his food without hunting for it. There are endless stories of the repentant cat. It is proverbial in the Book of Manus, one of the oldest known Indian texts. If you choose to cheat, you must accept the consequences and the responsibility, but the worst of laziness is that it often leads to unconscious cheating, especially if paired with ambition, for it leads to borrowing here and there until eventually you don't take any trouble at all, just like the cat who does not bother to get its own food. Butter Ears had either to hunt his prey or to play some trick. If you know what you are doing, it is your own funeral, and at least the repentant cat knew what it was doing, but people often steal intellectually and quite unconsciously. Lazy people have to become "catty" to live at all. Laziness practically forces you to dishonesty. People with a creative problem which they do not tackle are especially exposed to this temptation. I know many cases of people who really have a certain talent. Active imagination is a tremendous creative effort, and if people don't make it, they fall into the plot like Butter Ears.

Schiller says that play stands at the beginning of all culture because it is of no practical use and so leads away from materialism to more spiritual values. You find it in the games in the mysteries, and in primitive rites, especially the Dionysian mysteries. In *Psychology and Alchemy*,[3] Jung speaks of the Church's participation in the medieval carnival and of how, since the religious participation in the carnival and the *jeaux de paume* were banished from the Church in the Middle Ages, play and the Dionysian element are missing in our churches. He says that in early days even orgies were granted religious license so as to exorcise the danger that threatened from Hades. Our solution of the problem, he adds, has served to throw the gates of hell wide open.

Play is by no means purposeless, for it satisfies something very important. When the club was started nearly forty years ago, one of the first things Dr. Jung started was the Hallelujah game in which a knotted handkerchief was thrown from person to person and the person who fails to catch has to stand in the middle. It seems a pointless game, but it had an effect on the relationships in the club in preventing the members from being so intensive and forced them to relate on a primitive level. Playfulness is often at the beginning of creative work and is one of the best ways of starting active imagination. When people play with material and really enjoy doing it, then the thing is started in the right way so

[3]CW 12, par. 182.

that one can understand Schiller's statement. One can hardly overemphasize the importance of the playful element in the cat instinct.

To return to the pleasant, relaxed side of Bastet, which is playful in contrast to the highly serious mouser of whom Agatha Christie tells such a good story in *Come Tell Me Where You Live*, she says that they were taken to a house full of rats and mice, but that the Arabs assured them that a "professional mouser" was coming. It arrived and took no notice of food or people, unless they disturbed it by a noise, and in three days there was not a mouse or a rat. On the relaxed side, we need the luminosity of the cat instinct. Needless to say, the psychology of the person has to be taken into account, but the danger is not so great, because it may be that the person is far too strung up, too devoted to duty and taking life too seriously. A cat is a model for taking life as it comes and keeping calm about it. If a lazy person dreams of a sleeping cat, you may be pretty sure the dream will in some way end rather badly. This is a complete paradox, for relaxation is one of the most desirable things in life, but I think laziness leads straight to the devil. The meaning would be quite different if someone who was too tense had the same dream. You can generally see by the context which way it is meant.

INDEPENDENCE

Then we come to the last of our four threads: independence, which is a negative and a positive aspect of the real cat. The cat has the most extraordinary independence and self-reliance. You might say that Tefnut, when she left Ra in the lurch, went off to reflect in Nubia, but we have no evidence that she did. My garage man is very nervous and he got into a rage because he had done something stupid and Tefnut just went off to Ethiopia. The garagist is left completely in his negative Sechmet aspect. For the moment, you can only say that you have to go, and then, perhaps, Tefnut comes back. Tefnut, as Ra's anima, sat on his forehead and spat at his enemies. One must make conscious use of one's cat nature.

There is a story of a woman who was always so very efficient, and someone dreamt of her as a black cat which came into a room in which there was a mass of wool, which she mixed up thoroughly, having a marvelous time, and finally walking off with her tail held at a right angle. That is a picture of Tefnut of Ethiopia and her complete lack of responsibility. She mixes up all the wool! And then everything depends on how nicely you hold your tail!

Cat, Dog, and Horse Seminar: Lecture 3

May 10, 1954

In the last lecture, we came to the fourth and last of the cat and finished with the more negative, irresponsible side as illustrated by Tefnut. Lack of responsibility is a leading characteristic of cats. A dog minds terribly if you are pleased with him or not, but the cat doesn't care a damn, though certain punishments have weight, for purely selfish reasons, but the cat who minds whether you are pleased or annoyed is very rare. Dogs have strong feeling against people with evil designs. I read yesterday of a temple where dogs are used and can be relied upon to bark furiously at or bite people with evil intentions, while they are extremely kind and friendly to others. Police dogs also can, of course, be trained to know when people have evil designs, whereas the average cat would let its owner be killed and would settle down in the same house with the murderer, provided it was well treated. If a cat notices that you are in a bad mood, it just disappears, but not the dog, who is much more likely to enter into your mood.

The best example I know of this purely selfish and autoerotic attitude is in "Puss in Boots" ("Der gestiefelte Katze"). It is the story in which a miller dies, leaving three sons; to the eldest he bequeaths the mill; to the second, the donkey, and to the third, the cat. The youngest, annoyed at receiving something so valueless, determined to have the cat killed and have a pair of gloves made out of the fur. But the cat heard him and protested, saying he would only get a poor pair of gloves since his fur was not very good, and that instead the miller's son should buy him a pair of boots, in exchange for which he would help him. On receiving the boots, the cat walked off on his two hind legs. Now the king of the land was extremely fond of partridges, but the hunters were no longer able to kill any. The cat, therefore, seeing his opportunity, puts a little corn into a bag, takes it to the wood, the partridges dart in, and the cat seizes the bag and takes it to the court where he says that his master, a great count, has sent the partridges. The king is delighted and gives him a lot of gold. This goes on for a long time, the cat getting a sack of gold daily, until he becomes the tame cat at the king's castle. Then one day he overhears that the king and his daughter are to go for a drive, so he tells his master to go and bathe and, after hiding his clothes, goes crying to the king about his poor master who cannot come out of the water because his clothes have been stolen. So the king sends for some of his own clothes, and the "count" is able to appear at the court suitably dressed. The cat then frightens people into telling the king that some beautiful fields of grass and corn and lovely woods belong to his master, the count, and he himself goes to visit the real owner, a wizard, whom he flatters into changing first into an elephant, then into a lion, and finally into a mouse, when the cat eats him and promptly takes the castle for his master who marries the king's daughter and keeps the cat as his prime minister.

This story was first written down in about the early nineteenth century and appeared in Grimm's fairy stories, but it is a much older story and there are many earlier verions. There is no time to interpret the whole story, we must just briefly take the role of the cat who shows himself to be wily, completely independent, and self-reliant. It is unusual for an animal to be so extremely independent, but he works for his master as well as for himself. [An audience member made the following remark: It almost looks as though he used his master as a puppet.] In this story, the master keeps the good instinct as his adviser, but in many other versions, the master gets rid of the cat and the story ends badly for him. One is struck by the fact that, in not eating the partridges, the cat is acting against nature, showing extreme self-control. He really behaves like a detective. In most fairy tales, dogs tell their master what to do, but the cat here confides in no one and shows amazing shrewdness in hiding his ultimate aims. Brehm gives a good account of the way a female cat chooses its mate and then pretends complete indifference to it and even fights it furiously and is angry when pursued. The French have a saying descriptive of a woman capable of such action. They say, *Elle choisit celui qui devra la choisir* (She chooses whatever she will have to choose). If the woman showed her hand, the man would be in a position to make conditions, but by hiding her purpose and pretending reluctance, she keeps control. In the East, when each side plays the game of indifference, you can take from two to seven days to buy a carpet. We are inclined to think this human cleverness, but it really belongs in the instinctive realm. As far as I know, cats are the only animals that hunt in such an extraordinarily clever way, pretending, for instance, to be asleep so as to deceive their prey into thinking them harmless, thus demonstrating amazing control of hunger and greed. Elephants have a hard time protecting their young from a tiger, which always tries to eat the elephant calf in the first week, for later it is too late. An elephant will stay with her mate until she realizes that she is pregnant, then she goes off with another female (dubbed "Auntie" by humans). The two give their whole time to protecting the calf that is to be born and looking after it at the beginning. Oozies describe the way in which a tiger will try to trick the mother and her companion.[1]

The cat in "Puss in Boots" needs the boots to separate him from the earth, from *participation mystique.* A cat normally creeps about. One speaks of a "pussyfoot," but here we see represented the supercat which combines extreme shrewdness and cleverness with a human standpoint. It has something of the spiritual in it. We really enter here into the ultraviolet end of the scale. We had indications before, but the boots bring us fully to that end. It is actually the same idea as we met with in Egypt where Bastet is represented with a human body and a cat's head. Presumably the partridges, for instance, could not have been resisted without something between the animal and the soil. This gives us a valuable hint concerning our attitude toward our cat nature; we cannot change it, but we can give it boots, give it a detached and individual trend. This detachment, as we saw with Bastet, makes it more possible to deal with situations. I remind you of Niklaus von der Flue when asked whether it was true that he did not eat. His answer had the whole shrewdness of the cat in it and yet was completely human. The ingenuity of the cat here really comes far more directly from what Dr. Jung, in "Synchronicity," calls an absolute knowledge than from ordinary human consciousness.[2] The cat knows how to catch partridges that baffle every human hunter, i.e., we have an instinct somewhere in us that can enter the nature of the partridges and get the better of it. We have the same motif in the old nursery rhyme:

Pussy Cat, Pussy Cat, where have you been?
I've been to London to see the Queen.
Pussy Cat, Pussy Cat, what did you there?
I frightened a little mouse under a chair.

This is the same idea, namely that the cat instinct can enter anywhere, that human barriers do not exist for it, it can get to places where we cannot possibly find a way. This same instinct can also make the water, the unconscious, its accomplice. The cat hid his master there, while he played his clever trick on the king to get his master presentable clothes. I remember Jung saying in a seminar here that no one impressed people so much as the person who was detached and not caught by the things in which they fell again and again, the emotions,

[1]Lt. Col. J. H. Williams, *Elephant Bill* (London, 1952).

[2]CW 8, pars. 816–997.

etc. That the most impressive thing was to see somebody who had, so to speak, managed to wear boots and was not identical with nature. Again, Puss in Boots could enter the mind of the wizard and play on his vanity till he had him where he wanted him and could thus finally dispose of him. Afterwards the matter was simple, and his master had the sense, when he had reached the king's throne, to keep his cat instinct as his prime minister and adviser. In other words, he kept the contact with the absolute knowledge and therefore, though himself a simple peasant, was able to rule, i.e., through the extreme cleverness of the cat and his own shrewdness in keeping it, he was able to make a good job of it.

Jung has said that when we get to the point of trusting our instincts, we are apt to think that they can help us in everything, in all our daily life. But what does the Self know about taxation? We can only allow the cat instinct to help us where we really cannot see our way.

We have now, much too briefly and, for my taste, too superficially, worked out the four aspects of the luminosity of the cat instinct. We have looked at each from the positive and negative side. No doubt there are many other aspects, but perhaps eight are sufficient to give us an idea of the complexities and general lines that we require to interpret cats at all adequately in dreams or active imagination and give us an idea of how inadequate it is to dismiss the cat with a label such as "our feminine nature," or as the anima for men.

I really have not gone enough into how much the cat does represent the anima, and how much we have of the cat in ourselves; that would have needed a great deal more time. At any rate, these aspects give us some idea of how our cat instinct can help us positively and how, when uncontrolled, it can endanger us on the negative side. Puss in Boots made a good relation to his master who had given his last money for the boots. The wild hunter can help us as Ra, the tomcat, fighting the darkness and its vermin in our unconscious, or it can endanger us as the fierce wild Bastet, losing our energy in wild untamed emotions. It can bring us destruction if it is used as black magic—as the witch—or healing if the magic is tamed and used with a healing touch or purpose. It can relax us and heal our too greatly overstrained attitude as the pleasant Bastet, or make us lazy and false, like the repentant cat. It can lead us away into the desert, right away from our human relationships into a purely autoerotic isolation as the Ethiopian cat, or it can give us access to the universal knowledge and make us truly self-reliant as Puss in Boots. Of course, in this story it is the instinct which is self-reliant; by relating to that, we take over that part of our self-reliance which is projected into our instinct. I purposely left this story to the end, for nothing we can do for anyone is more helpful than self-reliance. I remember that Jung, in a seminar, said that we should realize what a help it is to our environment if we can become responsible for ourselves and not always try to find someone else. Another time, when discussing the parable of the unjust steward (the connection with the cat and the unjust steward is very clear), the unjust steward was praised because he did not collapse. He did not, it is true, behave very elegantly, but he was a going concern and by his cleverness kept his roots, kept his self-reliance. If we can do this, as Puss in Boots did, without losing relationship to others and even helping them, it really represents the summit of what relating to this luminosity can do for us.

THE DOG

Here we have a totally different luminosity or instinct. The cat represents an independent, almost wild, instinct that yet is very close to us. The dog is much more domesticated and is dependent on us in every way, especially on our society, and it therefore is much easier to train or educate than the cat. It could therefore be called an instinct which we can, to a certain extent, integrate much more easily and which would lend itself to development, even to a certain degree to assimilation. Both Brehm and Lorenz agree that there were domesticated dogs long before there was agriculture or before cattle were domesticated, and ages before the first traces of domestic cats. Interestingly enough, I saw a paper by Professor Hediger about foxes in "Sie und Er" this week in which he says that people used to think that dogs were descended from foxes, but this is not so. You cannot cross dogs with foxes, whereas dogs will mate quite happily with jackals and wolves. I am not so sure that this is the case with American native dogs, in fact, I have seen jackal descent denied in an American magazine. With *lupus* dogs, the attachment to men is to him as a leader, whereas with the *aureus* dogs the attachment is to a substitute parent. This is certainly true of the little French poodle which belongs to Dr. von Franz, whose attitude is purely that of a child to its parent. The dog is a social animal and loyal to its master. In the Christmas number of the *Saturday Evening Post*, there is an article by Sally Carrigher entitled "The Dog that Trained Me," which describes the relationship of a husky which is very enlightening as regards the *lupus* dog.

Whatever their original descent, Brehm says that wild dogs were originally tamed in their own countries. Probably, unlike cats, dogs were originally indigenous to the soil. Of course, through breeding and moving about they now come from all over the world and are very much uprooted. Brehm says that dogs very rarely sleep deeply. They certainly dream a lot. It would be interesting to know if cats dream. [An audience member remarked: Yes, they do!] Brehm divides mammals into sight and smell groups, because those are their two strongest senses. A great many dogs hate certain noises, but smell governs a dog's life. If the scent nerve is severed, a dog loses all relationship, even to its master. However, dogs with the flat, squashed nose do not smell at all well. They follow by sight and not by smell, and their eyes are very much better than those of most dogs. People say how nice it would be if dogs could talk. But how awful it would be if they really did. Think of what their conversation would be! What their neighbours had for dinner, and then think of the street corners.

Brehm writes that it is very difficult to say anything about the natural general psychic qualities of dogs because of the extreme degree of training. They are naturally cowardly and very seldom bite; they only do so if absolutely cornered, but they have been trained to be unusually brave and even fierce. He says that the innate quality at the bottom of their whole development with man is their docility and willingness to learn. Lorenz, in his book *So kam der Mensch auf den Hund,* says that it is a mistake to think that the educated animals are stupider than their wild forefathers. It is true that their senses have become duller in some respects and that certain subtle instincts have degenerated, but the same is true of human beings, and it is not in spite of these losses but because of them that man has risen above the animals. The breaking down of the rigid rails along which a great part of animal behavior is forced to run was the *sine qua non* for the development of a special human freedom.

Lorenz emphasizes that in training dogs one must never forget that they have no feeling of responsibility or sense of duty. The secret of training is to teach a dog that it may do certain things as a privilege, but it must always be "may" and never "must." If you can manage to teach in this way, they take an enormous pleasure in learning. Thus the secret of training actual dogs can be of use to us subjectively, in dealing with our own dog instinct, as we shall see.

Dogs are very maternal and, like cats, will take over the care of other small animals, even of their racial enemies, such as lion and tiger cubs. In the Zoological Gardens they are often successfully used for such purposes. But above all the dog is a companion. He is also a watchdog and, in arctic countries, is used to draw sledges and even here and in other European countries you often see them harnessed to small carts. The police and the army use dogs for many purposes and the large St. Bernard dog is employed for searching for lost persons and objects. They are also trained for use with the blind.

Dogs will eat practically every kind of food that humans eat. Cats are much more fastidious. Dogs are by nature carnivorous and like their meat high. They are therefore used in many countries as scavengers and even in some as corpse eaters. A traveler in Tibet in the twelfth or thirteenth century reports that human corpses were dismembered ritually by the priests and exposed. If birds, vultures, or eagles ate them, it was a sign that that person was going to heaven, but if the dogs or pigs ate them, then they would be reincarnated on earth.

I would like now to give the four headings of the main aspects of the cross hairs I propose using for our telescope of the dogs:

1. The loyal friend and its opposite, the betrayer;
2. The guide and hunter;
3. The watchdog and its opposite, the thief;
4. The habit dogs have of licking wounds and eating grass.

Healing myths are based on the last aspect. The negative side would be the devouring of corpses.

FRIEND AND BETRAYER

There is an enormous amount of mythological material about the dog, in fact, a chaos of overabundance which I have cut down recklessly. I intend to start with the first of our aspects, the loyal friend, which all dog lovers feel to be the most striking quality of the dog. It is interesting to find a widespread creation myth (particularly in Asia and Eastern Europe) that it was the dog which first betrayed man into the hands of the devil. I give an Asiatic Ugrian version. According to this legend, God created the bodies of the first pair of human beings and then ascended to heaven to see about giving them a soul, just leaving them as bodies on the earth and in the care of the dog. This dog had lived in heaven with God, who told him to be particularly careful about the devil. Now the first man had a horny skin, like our nails, and the dog a bare skin with no hair. No sooner had God gone away to see about man's soul than the devil came quickly, but the dog barked furiously, as God had ordered, and attacked him fiercely. The devil, being very clever, began to talk to him and tried to bribe him with promises of a nice fur coat, telling him that he was all right now, for it was summer, but that later on, when winter came, it would be dreadful. The dog resisted at first, saying that God would beat him, but some versions say that after three days—though the time varies—he at last gave in and sold man to the devil.

Then the devil spat at the dog, and he immediately grew a thick fur coat, only the tip of his nose remaining bare. The devil then spat at the first human beings and their horny skin fell off, but his spittle gave out so man was left with finger and toe nails.

On his return with the souls, God was furious and cursed the dog, condemning it to eat dung and be in servitude to man. In most versions, God gave man his soul, but in a Turkish version, the devil quickly blew his kind of soul into humans by the anus. In another version, this only happened to woman and "therefore the soul of woman is very evil, but her understanding is sevenfold" because the devil had used a seven-stemmed pipe for this purpose. (This might be very interesting from the point of view of the psyche of the animus.)

We will take up the one point in this myth which is always the same in every version, and which belongs in our subject, namely the betrayal of man at the beginning of his history by his later most loyal friend, the dog. Myths, as you know, represent archetypal motifs in the collective psyche of man, so there must be a reason why this one portrays just man's most loyal friend as the one who betrays him to the devil. We must remember that it was the beginning of the world, of consciousness, and therefore the instinct was *bound* to betray us, or there would have been nowhere for consciousness to develop. We would have remained in the harmonious ignorance of Paradise. When I told this myth to Dr. von Franz, she remarked that it was really the reverse of the story of the Garden of Eden, where it was man who betrayed God. He was the troublemaker. Here, it is the instinct that disobeys God and thus betrays man. [An audience member remarked: the devil persuaded the dog that God had not been quite fair to him in not giving him a fur coat.]

In order that consciousness may develop, a Promethean sin of disobedience is necessary and can come from either the conscious or the unconscious. In *Answer to Job* and in Dr. Scharf's *Satan,* it is very clear that the devil is the other side of God, so he can tell God better about his weaknesses.

We also find an interesting light on the action of the dog in Lorenz's book (p. 213). He says that all instinctive impulses of a wild animal are of a kind that will ultimately make it decide in favor of its own well-being, or of its herd, or pack. There is no conflict in the daily life of an animal between its natural urges and an "ought." Every inner urge is "good." Man has lost this paradisiac harmony. He says later (p. 214) that true morality, in the highest human sense of the word, demands spiritual achievements of which no animal is capable. The whole chapter is called "The Animal with Conscience." Lorenz goes on to deal with the undeniable fact that dogs do show a bad conscience often, and asks how that is reconcilable with their lack of moral sense? He explains it by the following story of a young zoologist. This man was an assistant at, presumably, the Zoological Gardens at Vienna and had charge of the young giant snakes and had to feed his pythons and boa constrictors on small animals the size of mice. He could either use fully grown mice or young rats. It is much easier to breed rats, and, therefore, he knew he ought to give them the young rats, but he had a peculiar feeling against it and continued to give the mice until the supply ran out. He realized then that young rats have a peculiarly helpless look, almost like a human baby, and that that aroused a certain protective feeling in him. He managed, however, to kill six and was punished for a whole week by dreadful dreams about these little rats in which they appeared every night, looking even more helpless and more human than they really are. They even talked with human voices and would not die. Then he learned that morality is not just traditional laws, but that it has also deep roots in deep instinctive layers of our psyche and that he could not afford to ignore deep feelings, however rationally right he might be.

This deep instinctive, undeveloped root of morality also exists in dogs, and Lorenz tells two stories to illustrate it. He had a French bulldog of which he was very fond, but another dog proved to him that it was his also. "Bully" was very jealous, and at last the two dogs had a most awful battle; Lorenz had to interfere with his hand and Bully bit his little finger by mistake. As soon as he saw the blood, Bully collapsed with a most dreadful nervous shock which lasted for several weeks, and he could not be persuaded to eat. For weeks he suffered agonies from a bad conscience. The fact that it was a mistake played no role.

Another time, the assistant went to a neighbor's house, and, as he was not wearing his usual clothes, the bulldog there did not recognize him and bit him in the leg. This dog, not being his own, did not get quite so upset, but looked at him in a most pathetic way and held up his paw the whole evening. Lorenz asked himself why this was? Neither dog had bitten before so it was not fear of punishment, so how did they know it was such a sin? Lorenz came to the conclusion that it wounded the same kind of instinctive feeling as the assistant had wounded in himself when he killed the baby rats.

This is of vital importance to us in understanding dogs and the dog instinct in ourselves. It is all a matter of which of these deep instinctive urges is the stronger.

To return to our myth, the dog there simply yielded to its stronger impulse, its longing for a warm coat. It seems like betrayal to us. For man it was betrayal, but the dog was true to its own nature. Evidently its feeling for God, its master, was not very developed, for the only objection it raised to the devil was that God would beat it, and eventually it decided that the fur coat was worth the beating. At my home, where the woods came up to the garden, we had two Skye terriers who were very much tempted to go off hunting. This was very dangerous and was forbidden. We had lost one already in the traps, so the dogs were always beaten, yet sometimes they would go off and stay away two days. They made up their minds that it was worth a beating. The female, who was very brave, would go straight to the man who would beat her, whereas the male dog hid in the rhubarb patch, but as he always hid in the same place, the man knew where to find him.

Dogs, which have a similar loyalty to the leading dog in the pack and will never stop fighting till he gives in, will only be loyal when they have such a strong feeling tie to us that *that* is the decisive urge, and even then we must not forget that they ultimately decide in favor of their own well-being, that is, they are loyal because the original elastic band to their home is attached to us, and therefore we are their center and most vital in their lives. This is a vitally important point to us, because we need to realize it fully to be able to live our life with our instincts and emotions. We may be able to do a great deal for abstract morality; certain people live their whole lives on this pattern, but they dry up, they repress their whole emotions, and eventually these will break through either with a terrific explosion, or the barriers will hold and the person eventually dies–actually or psychically–because they are quite cut off from the lifestream. You, all of you, know such people who look as though they had no blood left in them at all. If you say to someone in analysis, "What do you want to do?" it is amazing how some people will answer from what they think they *ought* to do. For many people, it is very difficult to get down to what one really wants, what is one's really strong instinctive urge in a situation.

There is a Russian legend that when God made men he made the common people of clay, but that the clay gave out so he made the aristocrats of dough. The dog sniffed at them all but ate only the dough. When God found the aristocrats missing, he suspected the dog and beat him or–in other versions–told his angel, or Peter, to get the dog by the tail and shake him, and each time this happened, out dropped another aristocrat! In other versions, the Poles, Lithuanians, and so on, take the role of the aristocrats. This is not only a betrayal story but has traces of the dog ancestor myths which we shall see are very common, i.e., in this case, the special people who had been in the dog's stomach. It also suggests the night sea journey, in a very primitive form, for the dog and not the hero takes all the action.

Freda Kretschmar, in *Hundesstammvater und Kerberos,* has collected an enormous amount of material in myths and legends where the dog is regarded as the first ancestor of a tribe, or even of all mankind. (I do not want to emphasize this too much as it is a common motif in creation and descent myths, and it is an honor which the dog shares with many other animals.) Freda Kretschmar says it is impossible to separate the dog from the wolf, jackal, and the American coyote in this field. In some primitive languages, there is even no separate word for wolf and dog.

Most of these origin stories are wildly irrational. Human beings are already there and one of them marries a dog—usually a woman and often a princess, though the sex is sometimes reversed, and then he is the first ancestor, even of mankind. This dog is sometimes a bewitched prince or becomes human, but more often it is only the children which become human. Sometimes, if a girl has refused all human suitors, the father punishes her by marrying her to a dog, or sometimes she runs off with her father's dog herself, to escape the incest wish of her father. But, as I mentioned before, this is not a specific quality of the dog, so I only mention it to show what a deep respect some primitive people have for the dog; they consider themselves honored in having him as an ancestor and believe him to be a worthy husband for a legendary princess. (The paradox is also visible here, however, for sometimes a dog husband or wife is an honor, and sometimes a degradation or punishment.)

As an example of the loyal friend, I propose taking one aspect of the Nordic fairy story, "Prince Ring," where the dog, Snati-Snati, plays a particularly important role. I propose only taking a few points which bear directly on our theme and not the whole story. Those who are interested may like to know that it is analyzed at considerable length in Dr. von Franz's book, *Archetypal Patterns in Fairy Tales.*[3] I will summarize the part that affects our theme: a prince, following a fleet hind with a golden ring round her horns, gets into difficulties which land him on a strange island where a pair of giants pick him up. They treat him well and only forbid him the kitchen. He tries to resist the temptation to look in but at last does so, and a dog there calls out, "Choose me, Prince Ring." When the giants are dying and he can have what he wishes, he chooses Snati-Snati, and when they are dead, the two leave together for the mainland. At Snati's suggestion they go to the king's court and ask for a small room. They are welcomed by the king but hated by the jealous minister, Randur, who incites the king to set Prince Ring impossible tasks, like cutting trees, killing wild bulls, recovering three precious objects—a golden suit of clothes, a golden chessboard, and shining gold which had been stolen, all of which had been stolen, all of which are now in the possession of the family of the giants. When he has accomplished these tasks, he can marry the princess.

By the extreme cunning and prowess of Snati-Snati, all these tasks are performed, and then the dog, at the risk of his own life, saves his

---

[3]See pp. 9ff.

master's life from Randur and brings the latter to disgrace. Then he begs to be allowed to sleep at the bottom of the bridal bed and is changed into a prince.

Like Puss in Boots, Snati-Snati takes the lead in this story, but the latter confides in the hero, whereas the former played a lone hand, very much in keeping with the related character of the dog and the independent nature of the cat.

The beginning of the acquaintance is very much like the beginning of a deep relationship between dog and man as described by Lorenz, particularly with dogs of wolf blood. It takes six months or a year for the *lupus*-blood dog to give its loyalty entirely to one person, and it very seldom changes. The first stage in this story would be when the decision is taken to do something about the unconscious and to give up the one-sided consciousness and turn towards the unconscious and find out its terms: enter the kitchen, the place of transformation. The man takes the first step in this case, and the original price of the dog is the courage needed in breaking the taboo of the forbidden chamber; then the dog takes the fatal step that links their fates by saying, "Choose me." This "choose me" is a frequent feature when one goes to buy a dog. My brother once gave me a Cairn puppy, but another of his dogs chose me, she always went with me, so, with great difficulty, I persuaded my brother to change. Then there is also the question as to whether the unconscious accepts *us*. We can do nothing in the process of individuation, or in taking up the problem of the inferior function, unless the unconscious is willing. If it is not, it will not send us any dreams and instinctive help. Here the dog accepts Prince Ring and begs him to choose him, so the development can begin. The third stage is the stage of fuller and sustained sacrifice. Payment has to be made again, and a bigger price than before. The ego will has to be subordinated to the will of the Self, and that is far heavier than the original price. Prince Ring remains true in choosing the dog when he is offered any possession of the dying giants. In the real dog, this represents the stage when we make sacrifices to fit him into our lives.

Cat, Dog, and Horse Seminar: Lecture 4

May 17, 1954

We stopped in the last lecture just as we were discussing the beginning of Prince Ring and Snati-Snati's acquaintance and comparing it to the beginning of our own relationship to a real dog and to the unconscious. We said that when Prince Ring went into the forbidden kitchen, this would be equivalent to our decision to transgress against the one-sided traditional viewpoint of our age and open negotiations with the other side, the unconscious, which is here represented by the dog.

When the dog calls, "Choose me," to Prince Ring, it is equivalent to acceptance of us by the unconscious, i.e., it shows whether it wishes what we wish or not. This is a stage in which we are more or less helpless and have to give the decision to the unconscious.

The third stage is where the unconscious has to make further and sustained sacrifices, giving up its rational will and accepted values, and subordinating the ego to the will of the Self. In *Psychology and Alchemy* Jung says: "To let the unconscious go its own way and to experience it as a reality is something beyond the courage of the average European."[1] Prince Ring shows this courage when he chooses Snati-Snati before any accepted value that the giants possessed.

It is interesting that in this story, as Dr. von Franz pointed out to me, obedience and humiliation increase. They go to the king's court at Snati-Snati's suggestion, but together, side by side. But in the third trial, the fetching of the golden objects, Prince Ring can only get up the hill to the giant's cave by holding onto the tail of the dog. This represents a place where consciousness would be powerless and where it can only accept the humiliation of being towed by the instinct. Now this task is the decisive one by which the anima is won, i.e., it is the *sine qua non* for a union of the opposites. Dr. Jung says that as we go on in the process of individuation, it becomes more and more difficult. While unconscious at the beginning, one can get away with a lot; but as we advance, the

---

[1]*CW* 12, par. 60.

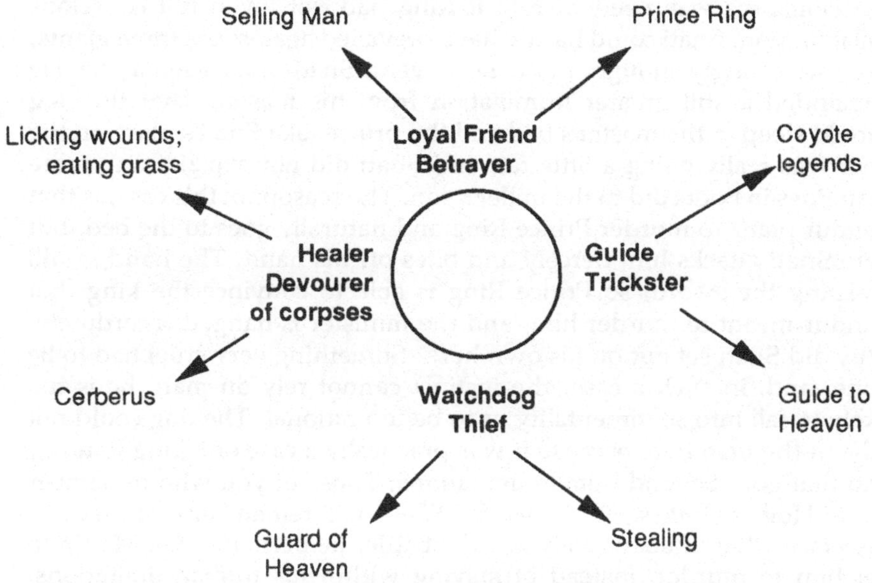

Figure 2. Aspects of the Dog

slightest deviation from our way is taboo, and often consciousness is just not sensitive enough to know when we do deviate, but our dog instinct knows the way unerringly and is a much more sensitive instrument in this respect. To go far in the process of individuation is a superhuman task. It can only be accomplished, as the alchemists say, *Deo concedente*. In *Psychology and Alchemy*, Jung compares the Christian attitude of throwing all our sins on Christ and being completely unconscious with the alchemists' idea that man can only be redeemed by his own very hard work. But even the alchemists say that this can only come about if God is willing, so in the end the Christian idea is accepted. Ring had to trust himself completely to his dog, he had to give up his last ego will, to humiliate himself and own his own weakness. But he had learned by experience that the dog could be relied on. We have to experiment until we know which aspect of the unconscious, which feeling and which instinct, we can rely on, and we have to be sure that it wants it also.

If Ring had trusted Randur, who was also an aspect of the unconscious, the shadow figure, it would have led to complete disaster. But consciousness was needed, too; if Ring had not given full conscious collaboration, Snati could hardly have prevailed against the three giants. Yet, interestingly enough, in the next event, Snati-Snati acted alone. He demanded a still greater humiliation from his master. That the dog should sleep in the master's bed and the prince take Snati's place on the floor was really going a little far, and Snati did not explain, any more than Puss in Boots did to the miller's son. The reason, in this case, is that Randur plans to murder Prince Ring and naturally goes to the bed, but here Snati attacks him fiercely and bites off his hand. The hand is still grasping the sword, so Prince Ring is able to convince the king that Randur meant to murder him, and the minister is hanged accordingly. Why did Snati set out on his own here? Something very cruel had to be done, and, in such a case, the instinct cannot rely on man, he is too likely to fall into sentimentality or to be too rational. The dog could not rely on the man here because it was practically a case of killing Randur, and that goes beyond human limitations. Those of you who remember James Hogg's *Confessions of a Justified Sinner* will remember that that was the place where Robert really lost the battle, he permitted Gil Martin to get him to murder, instead of staying within his human limitations. Here Snati takes the deed over and commits it himself.

I remember a girl who had no parents; she had only a sick aunt who was a cripple and extremely difficult and had an awful power attitude. The girl, however, felt she must go and visit her, since it would be too cruel not to do so, until finally her legs would not take her up the staircase, they just shook like a jelly. Dr. Jung, though before he had taken the point of view that the visits would not hurt her, said that that settled it; if the instinct was so against it, one could do nothing more about it; one must accept it. It is well known that instinct works by itself in producing frigidity if a woman marries against her instinct, or in impotence in a man.

The dog and instinct can afford to be more ruthless than the conscious could. If the conscious acted in that way, it would be almost forced to make Jesuitical excuses: doing bad that good might come, etc., but if the instinct does it, that is a *fait accompli*, and there is nothing to be said about it. If Ring had known in advance, he could not have let Snati be so ruthless. Of course, this is very dangerous, because it is really an invitation to make plots. To leave things one cannot manage to the unconscious is absolutely wrong. I am simply trying to explain that there are times when the instinct does act on its own. The dog wouldn't risk his master's life, and there he shows the summit of loyalty and willingness to give his life for his friend. Actual dogs, with the elastic band to the master, as Professor Hediger describes it, will also do this. According to Lorenz, this would be the strongest urge, because their own well-being depends on their master's survival. The question is, can we say the same of our unconscious? Of an unconscious that is fixed on the process of individuation I think we could. It is my experience that as the center is approached, as the Self slowly takes over from the ego, if the ego has really sacrificed its own way, sacrifices are also made by autonomous complexes such as the animus. In active imagination, it is possible sometimes to influence an autonomous complex in this way, to say to it something like: "Look here, if you kill me, our whole project will go on the rocks; you need the human being in order that you may be incarnated in this-side reality." This works sometimes, for after all, our bodies are the vase. Also the unconscious often acts on its own, just as Snati-Snati did, and can make us ill to save us from some folly. In active imagination, it may act suddenly where we least expect it: for instance, a woman was working on the country of eros ruled over by a tyrant and had tried every way to eject him but unavailingly. And then, quite suddenly, when she least expected it, he retired voluntarily and restored the queen he had deposed and imprisoned years before.

After all, individuation, i.e., the bringing of the eternal Self into reality, requires the life of the human being as a *sine qua non*, so we could say that it is absolutely true that our unconscious does go as far as Snati. At the end of the story, Snati-Snati asks to sleep at the bottom of the bed on the bridal night, and when his wish is granted, he turns into a human prince, also with the name Pring Ring. Evidently the fulfillment of eros is required to restore this dog prince to his rights. One could almost say that this piece of Ring's psychology had been lost (he had also been human before so that it looks like something which had been in human consciousness) and contaminated with chthonic contents, the anima, and the principle of eros, three things very much repressed in the field of Christian consciousness. Dr. von Franz says it is a very old fairy tale, written not so long after the conversion to Christianity of the Nordic lands, that is, somewhere between the eleventh and fourteenth centuries. She bases this on the fact that there is still no great tension between human consciousness and the instinctive world, as shown in the comparative ease with which Ring and Snati find each other and harmonize their points of view. In order to be redeemed, Ring must not only humiliate himself but also accept the anima. Then, suddenly, what he had regarded as a dog, turns out to have a spiritual content, i.e., he moves from the infrared to the ultraviolet end of the spectrum (to revert to the quotation from "Geist des Psychologie" given in Lecture 1) and the instinct, represented by Snati, reveals his archetypal meaning. It would lead us too far from our theme to do more than mention this aspect. By transforming into a prince, Snati turns out to be an instinct which can, to a great extent, be assimilated. The dog is much nearer to us than the cat.

Snati is a bewitched human prince, i.e., not quite a real dog, which we could never wholly assimilate. Snati is something lost to consciousness that was previously human. There have been times in history when people lived much closer to their instincts than they do today, and, therefore, much of the instinct represented by the dog can be integrated. In the original myths referred to briefly, this motif of the dog slowly becoming more and more human is extremely frequent.

GUIDE AND TRICKSTER

One of the best-known aspects in mythology is the dog as the guide of souls, usually to the other world, but sometimes also in this. We will deal with this important aspect, but as with most others, it is better to begin with the more negative side. We find here the dog as a misleader, or trickster. You will remember that I told you that Freda Kretschmar said it really was not quite possible to keep the dog myths apart from those of the wolf, jackal, and coyote. Lorenz writes that in the case of the actual dog it obeys its inner urge and to it every urge is "good." So in this aspect especially, it is really arbitrary to divide into negative and positive, and I am fully aware that it might be argued that the trickster brings about just as positive results as the dog as guide. However, in the dog, even more than in the cat, the aspects run into each other, particularly on the negative sides.

As Anubis in Egypt, and in many other places, the dog is very much connected with death. Therefore, we should expect to find him also on the side of abundant life. Especially in America, we find his cousin, the coyote, as a very erotic animal, who not only has every affair he can manage with the daughters of men, but also is actually the one who taught man the secrets of sex and thus brought about procreation and the survival of the species.

The Salishan Indian tribes in British Columbia and in northern Oregon and thereabouts have a great many myths and legends regarding the coyote, whom some tribes even regard as the creator and cultural hero. But here, as elsewhere in North America, he is a highly tricky creator, always up to mischief and using his powers to a great extent for his own amusement. For instance, the Shushwap tribe (a Salishan Indian tribe) have a story that he once changed himself into a baby and was picked up by two sisters out of pity for the poor, motherless, deserted baby. In the night, he secretly slept with each of them, and in the morning they were both pregnant. He is said not even to have respected his own daughter but to have got on to what he said was his deathbed and made her promise to give herself to the first man she met and, changing himself into a man, he met her in a wood and claimed her promise to her "dying father" for himself.

Such stories of the coyote seem to be endless among the North American Indians, and we find the same erotic promiscuity attributed to the dog in the Old World. In North Borneo, for instance, a tribe believes that paradise is situated on the summit of a mountain and that the door is guarded by a fiery dog who throws himself on every virgin that arrives at the gate of paradise, but lets every woman who has slept with a man on earth pass unhindered, for he considers her unworthy of his embrace.

The promiscuous nature of the dog is also very much emphasized in our common speech. To speak of a woman as a cat may mean that she is clever with men, like the cat who chooses her tom and makes him believe he chooses her, or that she is clever at playing tricks on other women. But often when women say so fiercely, "What a cat she is," you can detect a secret note of envy. But when a woman is called a bitch, it just means that she is promiscuous. Psychologically, she has fallen victim to a promiscuous animus and has lost her connection with the eros principle, her only reliable guide in matters of relationship.

Wild animals obey their mating laws whatever they are—some are monogamous, other polygamous, and so on. Most herd animals are polygamous, there being wild battles among the males in which the law of the survival of the fittest prevails.

Why should we find the dog and his cousin the coyote in myth and legend as such an especially promiscuous beast that he, particularly she, has become a byword for promiscuity? Dogs are more domesticated and really have their instincts more interfered with than any other animal, and their pattern of behavior is so much disturbed by living so near man that they have become unusually shameless, even perverse. One could say that the dog is an image for a rather unhealthy sexuality. The bull and the stallion, for instance, are kept for breeding and, though controlled by man, are given enough scope. But dogs are rarely kept for breeding and, unlike cats, they are not usually castrated. Thus, of all our domesticated animals, they have perhaps suffered most from civilization. Our own sexuality has suffered in a similar way.

I went to live in Paris for about two years as an art student when I was about twenty-seven or twenty-eight and was struck by the effect of the Quartier Latin in Paris on young girls who came there from America and England, particularly if they had been very strictly brought up. Some built the walls still higher and became even more strait-laced, while others in an extremely short time would go right over, almost becoming prostitutes. This was just after the first war. Very strictly brought up women are inclined to fall into a promiscuous animus, which is no doubt the psychological reason for the enormous amount of myths and legends where a woman marries a dog. Men tend to fall into the hands of a highly possessive anima who keeps her power over the man by continually projecting herself into different women. In the dialogue between Hugh de St. Victor and his soul, he asks what she loves best, and she says quite calmly that she has not quite made up her mind, that she either loses the thing that she likes through decay, or she sees something she likes better and feels bound to change, and there she expresses exactly that quality which gets in when this promiscuity gets the upper hand.

The connection between dog and trickster—mainly as I have given it to you in the coyote—also needs explanation. It is a totally different trickiness to that of the cat. The dog who sold man for fur and who ate the people God made of dough, and the coyote in the examples given in this lecture, takes his immediate pleasure, whereas the cat is like a master detective playing for a bigger stake with much more self-control. The dog trickster already contains an element of dawning consciousness. Such stories as that of the fiery dog or the affair of the coyote and the virgins either shock you or make you laugh, and then you are already not quite identical with the instinct. These animals show a kind of semihuman intelligence, pointing to the hypothesis that, with the dog, very much in contradistinction to the cat and horse, we are dealing with an instinct in between animal and man. The dog has become humanized, so to speak, that is, he is by no means a purely animal instinct. In my paper, "The Problem of Contact with the Animus," I talked of the woman with the anima figure she called "Archibald." He was most useful, a regular Admiral Creighton. She told us many years ago about this animus and of how he helped her, and we remarked that you could not really trust a figure of the unconscious to such an extent, particularly in regard to things of the outside life where you must make your own decisions. However, she would not listen, she was so delighted and gave herself more and more into his hands and became completely possessed by him so that what was originally very positive in the end became purely negative.

Thus the dog instinct has an unerring flair, but we have to be very careful not to let it advance into outer things too far. We must trust it in the dark unconscious, for it sees far better than we do there and its interests are usually identical with our own.

Coming to the dog as guide, particularly to the other world, the material is endless and comes from all over the world. I can only give you the merest fragment.

In Egypt there are two gods represented in old pictures as dogs: Anubis, who is represented as a dog lying down, and Upuaut (in Greek,

Ophois), represented as a standing dog. Anubis is a god of the land of the dead and belongs more in the Cerberus aspect, but Upuaut is a guide *par excellence*. His very name, according to Bonnet is already a proof of victorious advance in war and means the *opener of the ways*. He is so nearly related to Anubis (in Abydos, they are practically identical) that we must also mention that the latter goes beyond the shores of Egypt and, according to certain Greek writers, becomes identical with Hermes or Mercurius, who also has a caduceus, i.e., the thing which can open all ways. Hermes also has the Kynée, that is, a helmet or cap, in likeness of a dog's head, so that he is directly connected with the dog, not only through his contamination with Anubis. Hermes is directly connected with the Poimen and in modern dreams very often with the dog, in fact, I have had dreams of the dog that Dr. Jung has taken directly as the Poimen.

The idea that the dog can get us everywhere, especially to the beyond, is widespread. The Samoyeds, for instance, in North Asia (who also have a version of the "dog betraying man to the devil for fur" myth) usually gave their god Ngaa (death) the form of a wolf. When someone is very ill, they send for a shaman who places an image of the wolf at the side of the tent and then sacrifices the dog of the sick man (after leading him around the tent counterclockwise) and places the dog's heart on a pole. Then he kills another dog, praying as this one dies to the wolf Ngaa to accept this sacrifice in place of the life of the sick man. (They perform somewhat the same rite during a childbirth.) If these rites are unsuccessful and Ngaa insists on the life of the human being, they kill yet another dog on the man's grave and hang it so that the tail is pointing downward toward the corpse, with the idea that at the resurrection the dead man will hang onto the dog's tail and thus his soul will be safely conveyed to the South where he will find a second life.

In Further India they put the lead of the dog into the hands of the corpse, but the tail version seems to be the more usual. In Persia, in the Zoroastrian religion, this idea is still more developed.

In New Guinea there is a tribe that believes that pigs and dogs have immortal souls. There are two special dogs called Bigami and Vauri, who are the messengers of death and the leaders of souls. They come on the earth to fetch the soul of a dying man and are also dangerous, the belief being that while you are asleep, your soul flutters around, so no man of the tribe will sleep out of doors. The dog, as guide, can smell out the way with his highly developed sense of smell when none of our senses are any use, and he is so related to man through thousands of years of domestication that he will guide him as other animals with this acute sense of smell would not.

We must also remember that the dog is so much connected with death, the beyond, in mythology, and that the actual dog also is a sarcophagus for man in the many countries where corpses are exposed for him to eat, that he is really a dweller on both sides, the beyond and here. He is therefore particularly well fitted to be a guide from one to the other and even a mediator, for both men and ghosts understand him, so to speak. Dogs are also very sensitive to ghosts, and there are many stories of their being the first to realize that ghosts are around. In some countries in Asia it is believed that the dog will always show if there is a bad demon about. A doctor I knew always took a dog with him, and if the patient could recover, the dog would go into the room, but if he was going to die, would cower outside and run away. When it comes to the spiritual world, all reason and rational means come to an end and, like Prince Ring, we have to trust our dog instinct completely. Ring, however, had already been told where the golden objects were, he only had to accept the humiliation of being towed, i.e., owning that his own strength was quite inadequate to his task. Here it goes further, you have to venture into the completely unknown with only the dog instinct. In most of the myths, it is death, where there is no help for it, but psychologically when you venture into such realms you voluntarily have to face something so terrifying as death, or there can be no rebirth. You can have analyzed for a very long time and done a lot of active imagination before you meet this supreme trial. It even seems as if you were losing all you gained; "but if I go there, I lose all my psychological knowledge, everything I gained in analysis," one woman dreamed when faced with such a journey.

We find the same thing with the alchemists, for though they lay such an enormous emphasis on study, suddenly it is said: "Go tear up the books that your hearts be not torn asunder," and this even though they insist again and again on the vital importance of study and that all the books must be read repeatedly. Important though it is to the alchemist to know the right doctrine, he knows that on such a journey it is only a hindrance, and here it really is a fact that only an animal with a loving heart, such as the dog, can guide us in these dark places. It is the point where you have to give up everything that you have learned and go, only guided by your instinct.

WATCHDOG AND THIEF

Coming to the thief side, there is an amusing and widespread Christian legend, particularly in eastern Europe. I give an ancient Baltic Lithuanian version: God sent Adam to sleep after extracting the rib from his side and took a rest while he smoked his pipe. (In most versions he went away to get clay to fill up the hole in Adam.) While God's attention was elsewhere, the dog stole the rib. God rushed after him, but the dog saved himself by crossing a river where God could not follow; but he managed to catch the dog's tail, which came off in his hand, so God made Eve out of that.

We cannot possibly, in so short a time, go into all these eight aspects at all thoroughly and I propose dismissing this one part quickly as the thief is a well-known motif, and we already touched on it in talking of the lazy aspect of the cat and the repentant cat who cheated because it was too lazy to hunt.

As to this legend, partly a humorous dig at women, but also quite meaningful, the dog here really takes the role of the devil per se, the one who interferes with God's plans, and the fact that he goes over the river to the other bank–where God cannot follow–shows the duality in God which is so clear in *Answer to Job* and Dr. Scharf's *Satan.* He is like the other side of God, the one who is on the other side of the river. He tries to take woman in entirety, the whole rib designed to be Eve, but God just stops this and gets the dog's tail, a piece of the other side. God has to change his plans and make Eve more doglike and less human than he had intended. Women are nearer the instinct and more capable of dealing with the chthonic side than men. At the beginning of the last war, I had a dream that I was in Chichester Cathedral, where there used to be an unfinished chapel in which stones, etc., were kept. Here I met the devil and said, "What a mess you are making of the world with the war." He said, "Excuse me, this is not my fault, it is yours." I declined that responsibility, and he said, "Of course, I do not mean you personally, I mean women, because women can deal with the dark side and with evil and they don't do so, and so it gets into the hands of men who anyway can't deal with the dark. If the women won't try, then there are bound to be wars."

It is very helpful, however, that women at least grew up on God's side of the river, which prevented the other opposite from being too strong.

Perhaps the most interesting of the many myths and legends concerning the watchdog of heaven is to be found in Persia in the Zoroastrian religion. We hear in the Sad-dar, for instance, that to give bread to a dog is a good work, that one must never wake a sleeping dog on the road, and that altogether one should be careful to treat dogs well in order to ensure their help on the Cinvat Bridge which leads over the abyss to hell and to paradise. In the Videvdat (XIX, 30) we hear that a beautiful virgin guards this bridge and restrains two dogs on a leash. They throw down the unworthy into hell and guide the souls of the righteous over the bridge to paradise. We find these two dogs confirmed in the Bundahish and the Sad-dar (both Pahlavi texts). In the Bundahish, however, the virgin and the two dogs seem to be one large ghost-dog. At all events, in all versions, it seems to be certain that one or two dogs guard the Cinvat Bridge. A near parallel are the two dogs of the god Yama in Indian mythology, which also guard the way to heaven.

We meet the dog as guide to heaven in a yet more powerful position here. He practically occupies the place of Peter in the Christian religion and seems to have a lot to say, if not the actual decision, as to who goes to heaven and who is thrown into hell.

On earth the dog is more or less the possession of man, but here he practically decides man's fate after death. When it comes to the other side, we may be pretty sure that the decision of what is good and what is evil changes its standards. Traditional morality presumably gives way, as it were, to a deeper instinctive morality. One could say that what we call good, if it is against life, is rejected, and the same applies to what we call evil. I do not necessarily mean life on this side, which ends in death, but more a secret life manifestation of the psyche which is the vital and decisive point. This morality is really the morality of the process of individuation which aims at *totality*. The dog knows this morality better than we do, it lives itself as a whole being much better than we do. However the dog, actually, on earth, has a good nose for a criminal, for someone who has deviated too far from his own pattern. In Los Angeles, when I went to some friends of mine, I had to pass a Chow. I know and like Chows, and as a rule this one was amiable and pleased to see me, but if he growled or showed displeasure, I could bet that I had become inflated or that something was wrong. We say to beware of people whom children and dogs do not like, which shows the vital necessity of getting on good terms with one's instinct. You will remember that I quoted Dr. Jung at the beginning as saying that, for the analyst, it was vitally important to see if the instincts were with the emotions and that the latter were otherwise totally unreal. Yet this same dog can be a thief himself and even steal Adam's rib from God. This is the same paradox that we find everywhere. In the end, it is a question of whether we are at one with our instincts, with the paradoxical thing in ourselves.

Cat, Dog, and Horse Seminar: Lecture 5

May 24, 1954

The dog is not only the guard to paradise, as on the Cinvat Bridge, for instance, but also is perhaps best known to all of us as the underworld dog. Cerberus was originally god, the devouring god of the land of the dead and only later became the watchdog of Pluto. Cerberus is a real underworld god and cannot stand the light of day. As you know, the twelfth labor of Hercules was to carry the dog Cerberus to the upper world. Dr. von Franz tells an amusing story, namely that when Hercules carried Cerberus up to the outer world, he had never seen the sun, and when the first sunbeam hit his nose he sneezed, and where he sneezed foxgloves grew. Digitalis is a poison, and also a heart remedy, so here already we have a hint of the healing aspect. But Cerberus could not stand the light and Eurytheus could not stand Cerberus, so Hercules returned him to the underworld.

Homer mentions this dog, but without giving him a name. Hesiod first introduces him as Cerberus, attributing fifty heads to the monster. Later authors and artists confine themselves to a three-headed Cerberus which resembles Hecate, that dark chthonic goddess who prevailed over magic arts and spells. She herself is very much connected with dogs and was usually represented with them, being often thought of as with the dogs of the Styx and crowds of the dead. Black dogs were considered her favorite sacrifice. It was said that she was approaching when the distant howling of her dogs was heard, and the people fled, or threw themselves down on the ground, so as not to see them or be seen by them. Hecate's dogs were connected with the Furies who are supposed to bring madness.

We must remember that before it was discovered that rabies was the result of a virus and could be developed in any warm-blooded animal, sheep, etc., it was thought that the dog was the personification of rabies, which explains why it is so often connected with death and why we so often find them on that side.

Hecate is much connected with Artemis, i.e., with Diana, the huntress goddess, who is usually depicted with dogs. According to Hesychius, Hecate was sometimes even regarded as a dog herself. In later

Christian days, both the three-headed Hecate and the three-headed Cerberus became a kind of dark chthonic underworld compensation or mirror image of the heavenly Trinity, as Jung often points out. Cerberus, very much in contradistinction to the dogs of the Cinvat Bridge, is well known to have accepted bribes. Hercules, Theseus, and others got past him with honey cakes.

Freda Kretschmar points out that although it is clear that Cerberus was more than a mere watchdog at the door of Hades, there is no mention in literature that he ate the dead, which is curious because he is so widely known as a corpse eater. She also says that almost all the human figures connected with Hades have certain dog characteristics: for instance, Charon, the ferryman to the underworld, has fiery eyes and tousled clothes and growls suddenly so that he is even called the "human-shaped successor" of Cerberus.

As already mentioned, the lying-down dog in the hieroglyphic, Anubis, in Egypt, is also connected with the dead and is, in fact, a god of the dead *par excellence*. Freda Kretschmar brings countless other examples from all over the world.

We have already considered the dog in his aspect of guide to the other world, the one who can smell out the way in the beyond, and we must now consider him as himself at home in the beyond, and even in its not very reliable aspect as the watchdog of the underworld, open to bribes, and an extremely fierce guardian of the gate. This aspect of the dog Cerberus has to do with the angry instinct. If we repress the instincts, if we neglect to give them their meat, then they become a very angry watchdog between us and the unconscious and we cannot get in. You know that people who are on very bad terms with their unconscious often have dreams of angry animals or inferior men. That is the Cerberus aspect, the aspect of something neglected which then bars our way into the unconscious, and there is really no chance of getting through until the angry instinct is appeased with the honey cake. As honey is a spiritual food and is connected with poetic inspiration, it would mean, to some extent, that the way we get through is by using our creative side. You see people with a real block because they have neglected something. Very often people have to work on anything they can in order to give something of themselves. Honey is a natural food, but the honey cake is something made by the human being and therefore, at bottom, is a substitute for the human sacrifice. You have to give a bit of yourself in some way to this angry instinct before you can go or you will be kept out of the unconscious forever. If the instinct has been badly repressed and badly treated, it is really hell, and we must reckon with Cerberus each time we try to approach. Jung often says that when our problems are darkest, we cannot decide consciously, it is always the instinct that has to decide, unless we prefer an arbitrary one-sided solution which is not really a solution at all, but merely a repression of one side. If hostile, the dog instinct must be appeased and often, even when he has not been badly repressed, we have to act *contra naturam,* and then also we have to bribe our instinct to let us do it. Such an undertaking as entering hell to fetch up Persephone is dead against nature, for it means entering the realm of the dead while still alive and our instinct will tear us to pieces, like Cerberus at the gate, unless we remember its point of view and sacrifice something to it.

In the Eranos essays, which originally appeared in the *Phänomenologie des Geistes im Märchen,*[1] and which are just coming out in English, Dr. Jung gives a marvelous fairy story where he shows very clearly the difference between the witch (an attitude which is just trying to make use of the unconscious for its own purpose) and a real attitude of trying to get to one's unconscious and wholeness. In the story, the hero sacrifices the lambs, but the witch sacrifices nothing, and therefore loses one of the legs of her horse. Honey cake might also symbolize in its sweetness a kind of warm feeling attitude to an instinct that we have repressed or are forced to hurt by acting *contra naturam.*

HEALER

Coming to the healing aspect of the dog, we find this also in many times and places of which, however, the most famous is the cult of Aesculapius. Jung pointed out to me that it is very important that the wolf is the animal of Aesculapius's father, Apollo. (Aesculapius is the son of Apollo and the nymph Coronis.) As Apollo is regarded as such a shining and positive figure, it gives us quite a shock to find him so much connected with a wild and dangerous wolf, showing again the dual nature of the gods with which we are always confronted. But his own son, Aesculapius, who was educated by the famous centaur, Chiron, is the legendary god of medicine and, with him, his father's fierce wolf becomes the healing dog.

Although the fact that dogs played a role in Aesculapian temples is well known, it is very difficult to find any details. Freda Kretschmar lets us down here and all that she says of Aesculapius and his dogs is that there is a saga that he was suckled by a dog mother. (These legends of human children being suckled by animals are very common, for instance, Romulus and Remus, who were nourished by a wolf.) There is

---

[1] CW 9i, par. 384ff.

no time to go into this aspect, though it belongs in the healing category for it always saves the children's lives. I refer you to Jung's "Divine Child" in *Essays on a Science of Mythology.* In the *Revue Archeologique* for 1884, there are two interesting articles. The first of these is by a man called Reinach and is entitled "Les Chiens dans le Culte d'Esculape" where we learn that the word for dog appears on the pillars of a Phoenician sanctuary in Citium, showing that the dogs were on the temple inventory. Reinach then goes on to speak of two inscriptions on the Aesculapian temple in Epidaurus. The first concerns a blind child, Thyson d'Hermione, and says: "This child was looked after by one of the temple dogs and left cured." The second is even more interesting and reads: "One of the sacred dogs took care *with its tongue* of a child who had a tumor on its head." These inscriptions really prove beyond all doubt that the role of the dogs in the cult of Aesculapius go far beyond the watchdog and that they, like the serpent, actually took a part in the healing ceremonies and were, so to speak, the living vehicle for the healing power of the god.

In a later article, "A propos des chiens d'Epidaure" by H. Gaidoz, the author says that Reinach has proved beyond all doubt that these two cures at all events were brought about by the sacred dogs. He brings a great many parallels in other places showing the widespread belief that the dog has healing quality in its tongue.

In *Punjab Notes and Queries,* published by Captain R. C. Temple, it is said that certain illiterate Indians believe that the English kill dogs for their tongues, which contain a healing ambrosia, and they themselves allow dogs to lick their wounds for the same reason. What the Indians call "ambrosia" is referred to by the Venetians as "balsam." Gaidoz mentioned the same kind of belief in other countries, e.g., Portugal, Scotland, France, Jamaica, Bohemia, etc. A well-known French proverb says, "The tongue of a dog can be used as medicine" and a Breton proverb runs, "The tongue of a dog is healing, the tongue of a cat is venemous." Gaidoz also mentions the dogs licking the sores of Lazarus, which is, I think, the only positive reference to dogs in the Bible.[2]

Another reason why the dog is connected with healing is the fact

---

[2]Editor's note: At this point, a question was asked by someone in the audience, "What do you think about the healing in our instincts which is represented by the dog?" Miss Hannah responded, "It may be connected with the faithful aspect of the dog. If everything goes wrong, and we are completely out of tune with ourselves, something in us expresses warm concern for our well-being. It is almost as though instead of trying to satisfy our dependent needs from the outside, the power lies in ourselves to do this."

that he cures himself by eating grass and in many places is credited with considerable knowledge of herbs, knowing the right grasses to eat.

This last aspect of healing brings us into a rather different realm and perhaps the most positive one of all in this incredibly helpful animal, since it seems to lie in an innate healing quality in the tongue.

Yes, there is a source of healing in ourselves if we can trust it. People often dream of doctors and very often—if not always—such dreams can be interpreted on the subjective level as someone in the patient who knows how to heal. Such a doctor in ourselves would not be learned in all modern clinical methods—or only in certain cases—but would be more likely to be on the lines of a primitive medicine man. Through his healing quality, a dog in a dream could also appear in such a role. But it is clear that if healing is represented by a dog, it would mean that we must look for a cure in a humble place, as if we actually submitted to being licked by a dog.

The articles quoted above stated that dogs disappeared in the cult of Aesculapius long before the serpent, which was always a source of healing in the Aesculapian cult, Gaidoz thinks owing to the fact that dogs were so despised in Greece. In Aesculapian temples the serpent is also spoken of as licking its patients. The serpent would reach down to a far deeper level than the dog. One other fact that we should not overlook is that it is just in licking that this healing "balsam" or "ambrosia" lies. As you know, Jung usually takes spittle as "soul substance," a psychic substance, or essence. Therefore, we might say that the dog really massages us with the essence of its soul when it licks us.

SUMMING UP OF THE DOG

We have passed far too quickly and superficially through eight aspects of the meaning of the dog as he appears in myth and legend. These aspects—even if we had time to go into them properly—by no means exhaust the manifold possibilities or meanings of the dog in dreams or active imagination, but I hope that they may have proved how irresponsible it would be to hang a ticket around the animal's neck and say a dog means this or that. We saw him first as the betrayer of man to the devil for his own advantage and saw right away that we cannot afford to project our human standards of right and wrong onto a dog, or our dog instinct. To prevent our dog instinct from betraying us, we must learn its language here, so to speak, as it was learned in the dreams of baby rats fed to the pythons.

Then we turned to the more positive side of this aspect, in which the dog Snati helped Prince Ring to accomplish tasks that would have been far beyond human consciousness. We saw the summit of loyalty in Snati when he risked his life for his master and realized that our own unconscious is capable of a similar loyalty if we have a cooperative attitude towards it, as Ring had to Snati.

Afterwards we returned to the promiscuous and trickster element in the dog and saw how too much civilization has somewhat warped both our dogs' and our own sexuality and that the trickster element, although it is a kind of embryonic consciousness, bids us beware of too blind a confidence in our dog instinct; to let it lead us consciously is a totally different thing from allowing it to possess us as is always the result of a too *blind* confidence.

We then met the dog as the guide of souls to the beyond and saw his suitability for this task owing to his being at home in both sides. In psychological situations, such as symbolized by the night sea journey, we go as completely into the unknown as when we die and then—as we learn from religions and myths all over the world—the dog is widely regarded as the only one who knows how to find this unknown way.

We then dwelt briefly on the dog as thief in the Christian legend where he steals Adam's bone and saw him as the watchdog of the entrance to paradise, as illustrated in the Zoroastrian belief of the Cinvat Bridge. We find the dog here, almost in the role of St. Peter, and saw that it knows more of the morality of the process of individuation and wholeness than we do and that, therefore, we might expect him to know who has fulfilled the pattern of his life and who has neglected it.

Then we saw the dog as Cerberus and that a neglected and repressed instinct may well prove a Cerberus which prevents us from reaching our unconscious. Morever, we saw that even when we are forced to act *contra naturam*, we must never forget our dog instinct and neglect to give it some honey cake so that it will allow us to accomplish our purpose.

Finally, we came to dogs in the healing realm, particularly in the cult of Aesculapius and saw that there is a healing power in ourselves, but that it often needs great humility to reach this, just as it would be to submit to being licked by a dog.

THE HORSE

With the horse we enter into a different field again and one which is much more different from our two foregoing animals than the dog was to the cat. Except that it is also a domestic animal, it bears little resemblance to either.

Brehm divides the equine family into zebras, asses, and horses, of which only the last concern us here. Unlike dogs, who seem to have developed from jackals and wolves, the horse, per se, is found in very remote ages of human history.

The *Encyclopedia Britannica* informs us that wild horses were abundant in the prehistoric Neolithic period. Quantities of horse bones have been found near human remains of that period, pointing to the probability that they formed one of man's more important food supplies. The same reference asserts that "these horses were domesticated by the inhabitants of Europe before the dawn of history." But Brehm is more conservative in this respect, and opinions seem to differ considerably. It seems probable that horses were domesticated much later than the dog, and probably a good deal earlier than the cat. For the most part, our horses descend from European wild horses, although these were crossed with Eastern breeds, in England probably from the Crusades onwards, though there is no authentic account of Eastern horses being brought into England until the reign of James I when they are entered in the Stud Book. The Moslem invasion of Spain also brought a lot of Eastern blood to European horses. Brehm asserts that the so-called English thoroughbred has only a thoroughbred father.

Although horses are indigenous to America, according to Brehm they died out early and were reimported by Europeans after the discovery of America. The herds of wild horses in South America, Brehm points out, are horses which were originally domesticated and which have gone wild again. Such horses soon take on the habits of originally wild horses. South American horses have exactly the same habits as the wild horses of Asia and Europe which have never been tamed. Usually they are in very large herds, but within these there are much smaller groups consisting of a varying number of mares under the leadership of an old stallion. Both small groups and large herds are very shy and evasive, galloping away from danger, and their sense of smell and hearing seems to be very much more acute than that of the domesticated horse. Brehm emphasizes again and again that the horse gallops off if anything frightens it, or if anything is uncanny, or if there is anything it does not understand.

"Tschiffely's Ride" is an account of a man who rode from Buenos Aires to New York. He took two American ponies which had gone wild and which came from Patagonia. He describes them as immensely intelligent. One slipped down a precipice and caught on a tree, and he was able to go down and take off the saddle packs and the horse remained perfectly still without moving until they dragged it up onto the path.

Brehm points out that the horse, even in captivity, is one of the animals whose strongest sense is smell, like the dog. His hearing is also extremely acute. His sight is, according to Brehm, rather curious.

Although his eyes are so much larger than ours, they do not see stationary objects nearly as clearly as we do, or nearly as far, but they have an extraordinary sensitivity to anything that moves; a moving paper or a flying bird will make a horse shy, hence the use of blinkers. Brehm mentions also *der kluger Hans,* the horse who was supposed to be able to answer questions, and believes that the rider's smallest involuntary movement would be felt by the horse. If the rider did not know the answer, it is questionable whether the horse would.

Brehm emphasizes that the horse's natural reaction is always instantaneous flight. Therefore, it speaks for a certain psychic ability to transform and adapt that the horse has so largely overcome this natural tendency; one need only think, for instance, of the battlefield and the amazing courage of the cavalry horses. Brehm believes, like a good many other people, that the horse is not very intelligent—in the human sense of the word—and says that in its skull the space for the brain is very small in comparison to its long face. The intelligence of horses is a very controversial point. They certainly have a most remarkable extrasensory perception as evidenced by their ability to find their way, getting over difficult country, their high sensitivity to anything uncanny or haunted places. Even the gift of clairvoyance and prophesy have been freely attributed to them in many ages and places, but evidence of any reasoning power is rather rare. Of course, their extraordinary extrasensory perception and obedience to instinct often *seems* like reasoning, but if you analyze it—in my experience, at any rate—the cases which at least seem to be reasoning are very much less rare with cat and dog than with the horse.

Brehm divides horses into cold- and warm-blooded, or phlegmatic and fiery breeds, and even within breeds, of course, dispositions of individual horses vary enormously. The more their wills are broken, and the more we treat them like robots, the less independence and intelligence they show, but that is really because we cut them off from their instinct, and they form the habit of blind obedience which replaces the inner guidance, just as the white man replaces the inner guidance of the primitive. It is a fact that primitive tribes are inclined to lose their dependence on their chiefs and medicine men when government is taken over by a European country. Jung tells the story of how, when he asked an African chief about his dreams, he received the answer that they did not dream anymore now because the district commissioner knew everything.

The material on the horse is simply enormous, both the outer and the mythological. Even in a far longer course, I should be obliged to leave out many most famous examples. In the Bible, the cat is not mentioned at all, the dog has only a third of a column in Cruden's Concordance, but the horse, horses, and horsemen nearly two columns. One remembers, for instance, the important role played by the different-colored horses in the Revelation, but this is too long and too complicated to touch on here. An interesting book is *The Horse in Magic and Myth* by M. Oldfield Howey, but I should not venture to use it as a reference unless I was able to look up the material elsewhere.

We cannot deny that the horse is to a great extent a symbol for energy and libido (e.g., the power of engines is reckoned in this way) but it would be much too cheap to leave it at that. A much more general symbol is money, for that can be converted into almost anything whereas the energy symbolized by the horse is much more specific, perhaps we might call it temperamental disposition.

To find the cross hairs for the horse was most difficult, for they overlap even more than in the case of the cat and the dog, but the aspects of the real horse are the following:

1. Worker, bolter—the aspect of being fairly easily domesticated and the extreme ease with which the horse goes wild again;
2. Helper, victim (of man);
3. Imparter of vitality, of destruction;
4. ESP, tendency to panic.

WORKER AND BOLTER

For the worker aspect of the horse, I would like to remind you of the widespread myth that the sun god drives his horses around the heavens in the daily course of the sun. The number of the horses varies considerably, though perhaps four is the more usual.

There is an interesting Siberian myth which says that the sun is drawn by white horses, but that when it comes to the west, it is drawn under the earth by black horses and changes again at the east in the morning. Whereas the sun horses are usually white, Pluto's horses are coal black. On the rare occasions when he left his gloomy underworld and visited the surface of the earth, his chariot was said to be drawn by four of these black horses. There is the well-known parable of the soul as a charioteer and two horses in Plato's Phaedrus.[3] The horses and drivers of the god, Socrates says, are all both good in themselves and of good extraction, but the character and breed of all others is mixed. Man has a pair of horses of which one is "generous and of generous breed" and

---

[3]See *Five Dialogues of Plato,* Everyman Edition, p. 231.

"the other of opposite descent and opposite character." Later the description is fuller; he says,

> Now of the horse one, if you remember, we said, was good, and the other bad; but wherein consists the goodness of the one and the badness of the other, is a point, which not distinguished then, must be stated now. That horse of the two which occupies the noble rank, is in form erect and firmly knit, high-necked, hook-nosed, white-colored, black-eyed; he loves honor with temperance and modesty, and, a votary of genuine glory, he is driven without stroke of whip by voice and reason alone. The bad horse, on the other hand, is crooked, bulky, clumsily put together, with thick neck, short throat, flat face, and insolence, shaggy about the ears, dull of hearing, scarce yielding to lash and goad united.[4]

He goes on to explain how the white horse is obedient and the other completely unruly, always yielding to earthly passion, whereas the white horse would take us to a place where we could see the land of the gods, but—being tractable in contradistinction to the other—always turns to the lower things if the charioteer turns him that way. Most of you probably know Phaedrus, and the point is made here that the docile worker and the unruly bolter are taken by Plato as a marvelous image of the opposites in our soul which lead to our greatest difficulties. These are mentioned in the seminar several times. I will just give you brief references.

Visions, vol. 1, pp. 47 (Autumn 1930) where it is followed by the interesting story of black and white magicians where the anima first appears as a black horse, which would be of great interest to our theme if we had time for it.

Visions, vol. 1, pp. 151–153 (Autumn 1931) where the parallel to Plato's black horse is taken (vision) as the animus of women, also a very interesting aspect.

Zarathustra seminar, which I will quote: "To handle the good is no art but to handle evil is difficult. Plato expresses this in his parable of the man in a chariot driving two horses: one is good-tempered and white, the other black and evil-tempered, and the charioteer has all the trouble in the world to manage it. That is the good man who does not know how to handle evil; good people are singularly incapable of handling evil. So if God is only good, he is, of course, ignorant in reference to evil where he could not put up any show."

---

[4]Ibid., p. 241.

So really, at bottom, according to this parable, the art of life consists in being able to handle this peculiar, unruly horse, though, as a matter of fact, the completely obedient one also entails taking a lot of responsibility and knowing where you are going and what orders you have to give the horse.

On the one side, the parable of the two horses is a wonderful and exact image of the whole difficulty of man with his instincts, but, I do not know if it is personal, I have a somewhat dissatisfied feeling, perhaps owing to the fact that there are only three, and this parable therefore strikes me as a bit intellectual and optimistic. The optimism really consists in the fact that the charioteer himself is *one*. This is typical of Plato, for in his day there was no distinction between ego and self, and he often puts the ego where we would be quite sure that the ego was inadequate, and that only the self could function. However, it is such a marvelous image that I could not bear to omit it, but I also feel the need to point out that, difficult though these horses are, it is yet a little misleadingly simple, in that ego, shadow, and self are all contained in the figure of the charioteer.

Passing on to the second aspect, I must remark that though with the cat the negative aspect quite naturally always came first, this gives me a little trouble with the dog, but with the horse I feel forced to take the positive side first, i.e., that of the helper. I would like here to bring as an illustration the famous passage in the *Iliad* where the horse Xanthus warns Achilles of his approaching death. Xanthus and Balius, Achilles' marvelous horses at the siege of Troy, were celebrated for their fleetness, having been born by the harpy Podarge by Zephyrus, the generative wind. Achilles lent these horses to his friend Patroclus to fight against the Trojans but, after killing many Trojans, Patroclus dismounted from his chariot and was killed himself by Hector with Apollo's help. I quote from M. Oldfield Howey: "Xanthus and Balius were deeply grieved over the loss of their driver. They kept apart from the battle after his death, weeping, since first they were aware that their charioteer was fallen in the dust beneath the hands of the man-slaying Hector. They stood abasing their heads unto the earth. Hot tears flowed from their eyes unto the ground as they mourned in sorrow for their charioteer and their rich manes were soiled as they drooped from the yoke cushion on both sides beneath the yoke."

When Achilles next used Xanthus and Balius, he reproached them for having left Patroclus slain upon the field. This unjust approach unsealed Xanthus's lips or, as we hear in Homer's *Iliad*, caused Juno to endow him with speech, and he said:

> Yes, great Achilles, we this day again
> Will bear thee safely, but thy hour of doom
> Is nigh at hand; nor shall we cause thy death,
> But Heavn's high will, and Fate's imperious power.
> By no fault of ours, nor lack of speed,
> The Trojans stripp'd Patroclus of his arms:
> The mighty god, fair-haired Latona's son,
> Achiev'd his death, and Hector's victory gained.
> Our speed of foot may vie with Zephyr's breeze,
> Deemed swiftest of the winds; but thou art doom'd
> To die, by force combined of God and man.[5]

[5]A comparable translation can be found in A. T. Murray, trans., Homer, *The Iliad*, vol. II (Cambridge, Mass.: Harvard University Press, 1925), book 19, p. 367.

Cat, Dog, and Horse Seminar: Lecture 6

June 1, 1954

I would like to remind you that although it is not a label, the horse is usually connected with energy, or rather a kind of temperamental disposition, and that we can learn to domesticate and ride or drive the instinct, somewhat as we can the real horse. We cannot assimilate this energy—as we shall see—or only to a very limited extent, but we can get an attitude or relation to it similar to that which can be established to real horses.

We were speaking of the horse Xanthus in the *Iliad* last time, and I pointed out that he disidentified himself from fate, God, and man, and said that it would be by no fault of the horse that Achilles would shortly meet his death, but a result of "force combined of God and man."

The horse Xanthus, the personified equine instinct, teaches us here that it can carry us swiftly and faithfully, but that it, like us, is under fate and God, or in our language, under the Self. We can realize our energy, personified as the horse, and it can do a lot for us, but only if we live under the law of our being; beyond that, it can only warn us, *not* save us, for it also is subjected to the pattern of our fate, as Xanthus tells Achilles. It must not be overlooked that Xanthus ends his prophecy of Achilles' death with the words "God and *man*," for, very much in contradistinction to the cat, the horse symbolizes an instinct that, to some extent at all events, is in the power of human consciousness. Like all our instincts, it is not only ultimately in the power of God, or the Self. The libido expressed by the horse can, to a considerable degree, be domesticated, so it is altogether too much when Achilles rebukes his horses for Patroclus's death, yet this is something which we also do when we trust *too blindly* to our instinct. Horse and man are required to give this instinct its meaning.

VICTIM AND HELPER

Coming to the horse as victim, the mythological parallel would be the enormous prevalence of the horse as a sacrificial animal. This is true

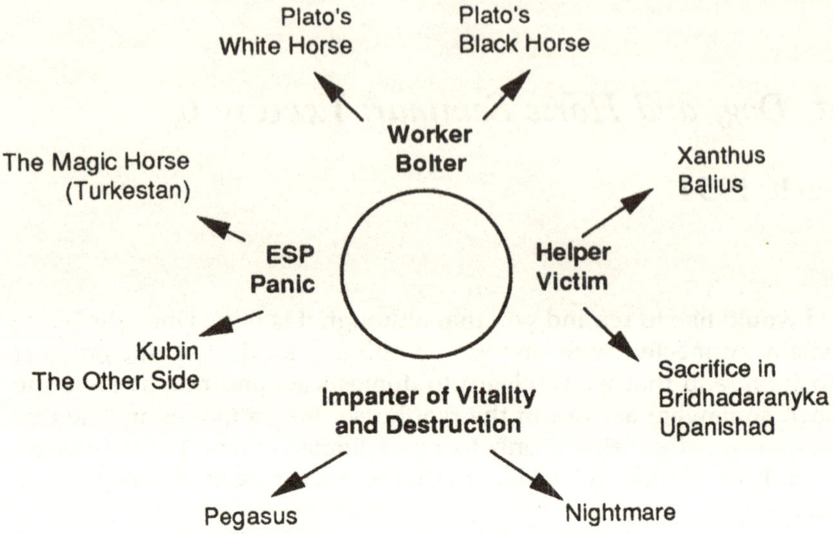

Figure 3. Aspects of the Horse

of actual, not only mythological, sacrificial animals. As the most valuable possession, horses were perhaps more sacrificed, at all events in certain places and periods of the world's history, than any other animal. They were regarded as especially acceptable to the sun and sea gods. It is interesting to find the same custom prevailing in many countries. For instance, many peoples offer sacrifices to their gods before crossing a dangerous stream. Heroditus tells us that when Xerxes (fifth century B.C.) led the Persian host and they came to a dangerous river, the river Strymon in Thrace, white horses were sacrificed before entering the water (Heroditus VII, 113). The Patagonian Indians also sacrifice a horse when about to cross a dangerous ford. Just as we saw that many tribes sacrifice dogs to lead their dead to the beyond, so it was the custom in many places to sacrifice a man's charger when he died. The remnants of this belief are still to be found in the British Isles. There is a story of an old Irish woman who, on the death of her husband, had his horse killed and, when remonstrated with, replied: "Do you think I would let my man go on foot in the next world?" In England it is still usual at a military funeral for the horse to be led behind the coffin with the dead rider's boots hung reversed on either side of the saddle. This is a custom of great antiquity and probably a remnant of the days when the horse was thus led to the grave to be slaughtered for the use of the rider in the world beyond. As an example, I quote the *London Daily Mail* of June 22, 1922, in which there is a picture of the charger of Field Marshal Sir Henry Wilson being led in this way in procession to St. Paul's Cathedral. Also in "Tschiffely's Ride," which I quoted last time, it is told how Mancho and Gato are led behind the hearse of their owner's great friend, Cunningham Grahame, in 1936. I can, in the case of a dog, quote my own experience on the death of my little Cairn. Out of purely hygienic reasons I decided to burn the basket and blankets she had had during her last illness, and afterwards I found myself thinking: "Well now she will be comfortable in the world beyond, she will have her basket."

Horses undoubtedly accustom themselves to other owners more easily than dogs, who might sometimes be really grateful for the revival of this primitive idea of sacrifice. There appeared in the papers recently a most interesting case of a dog in Tokyo who had been accustomed to meet his master on a tram at 12 o'clock every day. The master was killed in an accident and the body was taken immediately to the mortuary, so the dog did not realize his death, and for eleven years he met the tram. On his death a monument was put up to him.

Coming to the mythological side of the horse as victim, we will take the impressive beginning of the Bridhadaranyaka Upanishad as our example:

> Verily the dawn is the head of the horse which is fit for sacrifice, the sun its eye, the wind its breath, the mouth the Vaiŝvanara fire, the year the body of the sacrificial horse. Heaven is the back, the sky the belly, the earth the chest, the quarters the two sides, the intermediate quarters the ribs, the members the seasons, the joints the months and half-months, the feet days and nights, the bones the stars, the flesh the clouds. The half-digested food is the sand, the rivers the bowels, the liver and the lungs the mountains, the hairs the herbs and trees. As the sun rises, it is the forepart, as it sets, the hindpart of the horse. When the horse shakes itself, then it lightens; when it kicks, it thunders; when it makes water, it rains; voice is its voice.
>
> Verily Day arose after the horse as the [golden] vessel, called Mahiman [greatness], which [at the sacrifice] is placed before the horse. Its place is in the eastern sun. The Night arose after the horse as the [silver] vessel, called Mahiman, which [at the sacrifice] is placed behind the horse. Its place is in the western sea. Verily, these two vessels [or greatnesses] arose to be on each side of the horse.
>
> As a racer he carried the Devas, as a stallion the Gandharvas, as a runner the Asuras, as a horse men. The sea is its kin, the sea is its birthplace.

Jung says, in *Symbole der Wandlung* (the new English edition replaces the original *Psychology of the Unconscious*, but I have made the following translation directly from the German), that we find the horse here as a symbol of time, but also as the whole world.[5] Later he says that in this Upanishad:

> The horse symbol contains the whole world in itself, its relations and cradle are the sea, the mother, equal to the world soul. Just as Aion represents the libido in "being swallowed," i.e., in the stage of death and rebirth, so also here the sea is the cradle of the horse, that is, the libido, is in the mother, that is the Unconscious, dying and being resurrected.[6]

Later he returns to this again and says:

> As Doussen remarks, the sacrifice of the horse has the meaning of a *renunciation of the universe.* When the horse is sacrificed, the world is as it were sacrificed and destroyed, a train of thought which also presented itself to Schopenhauer. In the above text the horse stands between two sacrificial bowls, it comes from the one and goes to the other as the sun goes from morning to evening. In that the horse is the riding and working animal of man and that the latter even measures energy in terms of horsepower, so it represents a sum of energy which is at his disposition. We saw above that it is necessary to sacrifice the libido which adheres to the mother in order to produce the world; here (in the Upanishad) the world is put an end to by the renewed sacrifice of the same energy which first belonged to the mother, and then flowed into the world. The horse can be used here appropriately for, as we saw above, it has a manifold relation to the mother. By the sacrifice of the horse, a phase of introversion can again be produced which is similar to that of the creation of the world. The position of the horse between the two vessels which represent the productive and devouring aspects of the mother, point towards the image of life contained in the egg so that the vessels are meant to surround the horse. This is proved later in the same Upanishad (3,3).[7]

Jung continues with this passage, but time forces me to condense unwarrantably, as I only give you one more sentence of his interpreta-

---

[5] CW 5, par. 425.

[6] CW 5, par. 426.

[7] CW 5, par. 658.

tion: "As this text (the part omitted) says: those who sacrifice the horse come into the smallest fissure between the shells of the world egg at that place where they are both united and separated."[8]

The sacrifice of the libido in the mother usually takes place unconsciously as a young man's libido passes out into the world as he grows up. Therefore, we could say that the sacrifice of the outer libido in the world, symbolized here as the horse, is the first *conscious* sacrifice of libido for the sake of introversion.

Dr. Jacobsohn takes the Ka in his lectures on the Egyptian religion as the aspect of the Self that is effective in the world, whereas the Ba is the aspect of the Self that withdraws into introversion. The sacrifice of the horse is the moment of turning from the outer to the inner. Although I want to take the nightmare aspect later, I must just mention here that it also represents such a turning inwards of the libido, but happening to us unconsciously in sleep, that is, involuntarily, but I will return to this later.

I would like to give here a piece of modern material which exactly fits the situation. It is the first dream when she came into analysis of a French woman living in the west of America. This woman was about forty-two. She had had a fairly successful business life and a less successful marriage. She was exceedingly extraverted but came from a very religious background so that something in her life was considerably in revolt against the empty life she was leading. She dreams that animals are being sacrificed. A horse is on the altar. She sees that it is not dead. She is very upset and signs to the sacrificer, a man, and he approaches with a large syringe to give the horse its *coup de grace*, but the horse raises its head and stares straight into the man's eyes, and the dream ends while they are motionless, looking at each other.

We find an interesting parallel to man and horse looking into each other's eyes in the medieval *Chansons de Geste* (epic chronicles, a group of which centers around Charlemagne, ca. 742–814). Bayard was the famous demon horse of Aymon of Dordogne who managed to give Charlemagne a peck of trouble owing to the horse's magic powers. On his death, Aymon left Bayard to his youngest son, Renaud, whom Bayard served faithfully, but later the four sons, finding themselves at the mercy of the emperor, purchased his forgiveness by handing over the demon horse to be put to death. The emperor, considering that all the trouble had come through the horse, weighted his hooves with lead and had him driven into the Seine to drown. Twice Bayard rose to the

---

[8]CW 5, par. 659.

surface and met his master's eyes in a look of agonizing appeal, but as he rose for the third time, his stricken master Renaud, his heart breaking, had fallen in anguish to the ground and—missing his master's eyes—the horse sank for the last time. Renaud, maddened by the torture of his faithful friend, tore up the pardon of the emperor and threw it at his feet, and tradition asserts that he gave up the world and went on a crusade and then became a hermit known for his holy life.

This story is quite interesting to us as it illustrates very vividly in medieval legend exactly the process which Jung attributes to the sacrifice of the horse, marking a complete change from an extraverted worldly life to the inner life of a hermit. Those of you who go to Dr. von Franz's lectures on Niklaus von der Flue will remember the role that the horse played in a vision of the Swiss saint before he also left the world and settled in the Ranft.

To return to our modern dreamer, we must consider what the unconscious might be trying to tell her. She was just past the middle of life, so presumably it was time for her to withdraw her libido from the world, though not in the sense of becoming a hermit. She is called upon to sacrifice something. As you know, we possess nothing really unless we have sacrificed it, an idea difficult to understand unless one has had the experience. (I refer you to what Jung says about that aspect of sacrifice in his lecture on the Mass, which is now coming out in English.)[9] The dreamer was, in a way, "staring at" the things she wanted. Now if you consciously "stare at" things, they never come into reality. I remember the case of a girl who had been brought up by her mother to marry, so she "stared at" that possibility in the case of every eligible man who came near her. She got on all right with men as long as they were not marriageable. It was only when she was over forty, and in analysis, that she faced the possibility of never marrying. Later she married a man who said he had wanted this for a long time, but for some reason had found it impossible.

The dreamer evidently shuns pain, but the horse knows that the pain is necessary and instead of welcoming the syringe, he exposes the man (the animus who does first what she must do later) to looking into the eyes of the animal. Jung says of the eyes of an animal, when they come in the Visions (vol. 1, p. 62):

> This is the first vision where she is quite positively stung; she has been more or less sightseeing, but here it gets under her skin. She made a picture of the face, it is that of an

---

[9]CW 11, par. 307.

> animal, a dark hairy face with the melancholy eyes of a beast. What really happened was they not only traveled back to ancient Greece but went even further, the animals led her back even into the animal age. You remember that the purpose of the Dionysian mysteries was to bring people back to the animal; not to what we commonly understand by that word, but to the animal within. She looks directly into the eyes of an animal, and they are full of woe and beauty because they contain the truth of life, an equal sum of pain and pleasure, the capacity for joy and the capacity for suffering. The eyes of very primitive and unconscious men have the same strange expression of a mental state before consciousness, which is neither pain nor pleasure; one doesn't know exactly what it is, it is most bewildering, but undoubtedly she here sees into the very soul of the animal, and that is the experience she should have. Otherwise she is disconnected from nature.

Our dreamer also has to look into the truth of life, into truth and beauty, into the experience of which her superficial life is robbing her. "Looking into the eyes" would be establishing psychic contact, which the dream says can only be achieved through sacrifice. From other dreams, it was evident that she had been living completely at the infrared end of the scale and here she is offered the opportunity of seeing the meaning, moving towards the ultraviolet end and learning something of the archetypal image of the instinct she has just lived blindly.

The nightmare is closely related to the sacrificial aspect. Oldfield Howey quotes some modern instances of nightmare from the contemporary press and gives the following extract from the *Daily Express* of February 5, 1920:

> Death during nightmare, the problem raised at the inquest on a convict who died in his sleep, was much discussed in medical circles yesterday. "There is nothing improbable in the suggestion of death caused by nightmare," said Dr. Welby Fisher of Harley Street, formerly a member of the staff of St. George's Hospital, to a *Daily Express* representative. "Victims of these unpleasant sensations always experience difficulty in breathing. With persons suffering from angina pectoris, the struggle for breath during nightmare would cause death. A normally healthy person would not be likely to die of these nocturnal terrors, but one who is physically weak would lack the power to withstand the terrible strain. Nightmare is more common with children than with adults, but I have never known a child to die in these circumstances. Grown up people who are subject to a recurrence of these distressing symptoms should exercise the greatest care. . .as neglect of the simple rules of health may bring the nightmare of death.

The *Express* further comments on this in a leading article:

> The dictionary interpretation of a nightmare is an incubus or evil spirit that oppresses people during sleep. . . .Whatever the cause, there is no question that the effects of a nightmare leave their mark on the human brain for a lifetime. The question is now raised whether such visions may not be the cause of many sudden deaths which occur during sleep. Leading medical authorities agree that this is a very frequent explanation in the case of persons suffering from extreme physical exhaustion.

Jung, in *Symbole der Wandlung*,[10] says that the Germanic root of the word *mare* is *mar* which means dying, so it is interesting to find a discussion in a modern newspaper seriously considering that nightmare can even be a cause of death. Jung says that lamias are typical nightmares and abundant evidence points to their feminine character. We hear everywhere that they ride their victims. Their counterpart is the ghostly horse that carries away its riders at a mad gallop. Oldfield Howey has collected a lot of legends where the rider is never heard of again.

We do not have the time here to go into the subject more deeply, as Jung does. He particularly connects the nightmare with getting the energy back from the mother and later from the world. In the notes to this page, he refers to other literature on the same subject. The point I want to make is that if nothing is done to free this libido, it becomes regressive and sits on one's chest like a nightmare, or it carries one away from the world like the ghostly horse—a wonderful picture of being possessed by the animus and isolated by him far from human contact, that is, of course, in the psychology of women.

From its connection with the lamia, the nightmare also represents the anima in her most possessive form. I must remind you of the origin of the word *lamia*. The Queen of Libya, Lamia, had a love affair with Zeus and the jealous Hera managed to prevent Lamia from ever bringing a living child into the world, which made her dreadfully bitter and she became the bloodthirsty destroyer of every child she could reach. She also represents a particularly cold-blooded form of anima, enticing young men into her embrace so that she might feed on their life and young blood. I would also remind you of Keats's "Lamia." Who can say how much this demon anima had to do with his death in his twenty-sixth year? Again, there is his haunting ballad, "La Belle Dame Sans Merci," one of the most terrible anima poems in the English language;

---

[10] *CW* 5, par. 370ff.

the anima in her deathly aspect without her compensating activity of entangling a man in the world. Keats is a phenomenon himself, which we cannot go into here, and if we did, it would really belong more in the Pegasus aspect.

At bottom one might perhaps say that the horse in his nightmare aspect is intimately connected with the problem of the anima for men, and the animus for women, and this is perhaps the simplest way of expressing the necessity of sacrificing one's horse libido, for without this one will remain possessed by these figures in their most negative and possessive aspect. They will literally suffocate one or gallop away with one, so that leaves one's whole individual pattern unlived.

IMPARTER OF VITALITY AND DESTRUCTION

The way out of the deadlock of the nightmare is obviously connected with the creative and is again symbolized by a horse, the famous Pegasus. This winged horse of Greek fable is said to have sprung from the trunk of the gorgon Medusa when Perseus cut off her head, a most clear symbol of what is produced by the sacrifice of the mother in her petrifying nightmare aspect.

The sea god Poseidon was said to be the father of Pegasus, a god very much connected with horses. Most unfortunately, we shall have to leave out that aspect as we have no time for it. Bellerophon was said to be the first mortal who rode Pegasus. According to some accounts, he was also a son of Poseidon and therefore the brother of his own horse. On Poseidon, Bellerophon slew Chimaera. Chimaera was originally a monster, so Dr. von Franz tells me, whose forepart was a lion, whereas the hind part was a dragon and the middle part a woman. We must resist this fascinating symbolism and only point out that the name of this monster, Chimaera, has become the common word for mere wild fancies with no foundation, for delusions. That it was just this monster that Bellerophon had to slay while riding on the horse that had sprung from the destroyed gorgon Medusa is another marvelous symbol, not only of the necessity for slaying the mother but also for the fantastic plans and unrealities connected with her. Otherwise expressed, we could say that the wrong kind of active imagination must be slain before Pegasus can come into his own as the real creative libido.

Bellerophon, indeed, himself came to a bad end from his ambitious attempt to ascend to the heavens on Pegasus. The angry gods send a gadfly to sting him so that he shied and threw Bellerophon to the earth where, lamed and blinded, he became a wanderer, separated from Pegasus for the rest of his life. Again, here, we see a typical danger of creative libido: it tries to rise too high and thus lames itself fatally. We will return to this aspect later.

Many of you will remember that Pegasus was mentioned in a very interesting way in Jung's Visions seminars not only as the inspiration of the poet, but as a new ruling astrological principle. He says:

> The interesting thing is that Pegasus is entirely symbolic, it is no longer a human principle, it is quite decidedly the animal principle. We would say that the horse is a libido symbol, it is the animal part of man which he is pulling himself up upon, which he is riding, and thus it becomes winged, it is divine; it is not only an ordinary animal, it is a divine animal. So it would mean a time in which man discovers that the real guiding principle is the living libido. And that would be represented by a square. How people could ever imagine that Pegasus should be represented by that square is a miracle to me, but they did.

In this age, in other words, the three has been superseded by the four, symbolized by the square of Pegasus. It is really interesting that this winged horse which, as with Bellerophon, is connected with human ambition, can lead to inflation, should be just the one to supply the missing fourth. Pegasus is himself a symbol that united the opposites, a chthonic animal, absolutely of the earth and yet with wings belonging to the spiritual realm. He is a symbol similar to the famous winged serpent in the Aztec religion. He unites the chthonic and the spiritual, therefore he leads toward wholeness, the quaternity and the square. Thus, if we are to ride Pegasus at all, we need to do so with the *utmost* humility and all ambitious plans and high flights are taboo and would lead to the fate of a Bellerophon.

Personally, I should also say that Pegasus, regarded as true creative inspiration, in spite of his high flights, is just the one to bring us down to earth, for if we have to *produce* something, we are soon checked in our high flights. Anyone who has tried to reduce a vision, for instance, to paint or words knows the utter despair that rises in one when confronted with the hopeless task of producing anything satisfactory. The creative libido of Pegasus is only dangerous if we allow it to divorce us from reality. If we succeed in combining it with *work*, it brakes itself for, as we have seen, the square of Pegasus is connected with the totality, the hardest job there is, whether attempted by a creative artist or in making real the process of individuation.

In bad cases of inflation, one often meets the symbol of an eagle. In *Confessions of a Justified Sinner* by James Hogg, just before he fell into the hands of Gil Martin, Robert says that he felt as if he were an eagle flying above the world and looking down upon groveling mankind. With Pegasus, we are not dealing with a bird but a horse with all a horse's qualities which cannot be ignored just because he also has wings. The Bellerophon myth is really an excellent picture of creative libido. After the first battle with the Chimaera is won and you are able to use your libido creatively, a second battle has to be fought against overambition, which is particularly dangerous when combined with laziness. There comes the temptation to ignore one's earthly limits, to let the monster Chimaera revive and indulge in high flights of unreal fantasy, joining the gods, as Bellerophon tried to do, which will lead to a fatal fall and to a lame or blind existence. But if you do not forget that your horse is flesh and blood and humbly keep to your own limitations, above all to the hard work which is a main characteristic of the horse, the catastrophe of Bellerophon can be avoided.

PANIC AND ESP

This aspect naturally is considerably connected with the nightmare. One of the greatest dangers of nightmare is that it will result in panic, for everything depends on how the content is taken. If it can be accepted with some degree of self-control, a nightmare may even turn out to be a blessing in disguise. Jung once said to me, from a dream I had had, that there was really only one danger in the unconscious and that was the danger of panic. If that could be avoided, then it was difficult but possible to find one's way through every other difficulty that confronted you. The great danger is that you get infected with the panic of the horse.

The horse is particularly exposed to this danger, for, as Brehm points out, his natural reaction in the wild state is instantaneous flight. Not that this is necessarily panic; it can—in the wild state—be an orderly retreat, a sort of "he who fights and runs away, lives to fight another day." But, as his contact with man has so largely robbed him of his natural reaction, it has become repressed, like so many of our own human instincts, and when it breaks through, it is really a terrifying thing. A badly frightened horse, that takes the bit between his teeth and bolts, was the only thing in my riding days that frankly scared me stiff.

It is difficult to say where panic ends and madness begins, but they are very close. In fact, when in the grip of a wild panic, one might almost say that the sanest person is temporarily mad.

A literary example of such a state, often mentioned by Jung, is in a book written shortly before or during the 1914-1918 war: *The Other Side* by a German called Alfred Kubin. Unfortunately, there is no English translation. The book leaves a nasty taste in your mouth, and Jung says of it that it is a description of the collective unconscious in which the man Kubin is almost caught and that he only just escaped a psychosis. I should mention that Kubin was really an artist. He illustrates this fantastic novel himself. The hero of the fantasy, also an artist, is tempted by a large sum of money to join an old school friend who has established a so-called "dream state" a day or two's journey beyond Samarkand (north of Afghanistan in Russian Central Asia). Alternatively jubilant and terribly depressed, he and his wife accomplish the long journey by Constantinople and the Caspian Sea in *outer conditions* as far as Samarkand, but from there on they reach the "other side," this dream state, where the sun never shines and there is little or no change in the seasons.

Almost at once they realize that something is badly wrong, but for two years they have no idea what. Then—driven by the nervous agonies of his wife—the hero goes to investigate the noises that are driving her mad and finds that they are due to an almost starved and maddened white horse which is galloping around in a wild panic, imprisoned in the cellars beneath the town. Jung describes this horse as "a thing that does not find its way out, life that got lost in the tombs of the collective unconscious and went mad." He also described it as " the personification of panic," a riderless horse, a piece of libido that should be ridden by man but is lost here in the underground cellars.

Naturally this is an extreme case but it illustrates very vividly the great danger of not being in connection with our horse instinct. If we can domesticate our horse power, our temperamental disposition, we can ride or drive it, it is our fruitful helper, even in our most difficult situations, but if we starve or repress it, as Kubin evidently had done, we shall only meet it in the form of a wild panic when it can endanger our life and, still worse, our reason.

It is no chance that Kubin was an artist, for this danger is particularly acute where there is a creative problem. If we fail to meet the demands of the creative spirit within us, if we do not use our Pegasus, in however humble a form he may present himself, to the utmost of our ability, whether in active imagination or outer creative work—we repress him, and then he inevitably becomes, sooner or later, this white horse imprisoned in the cellars which at first will only be realized as curious ghostly noises coming from one knows not where, vague terrors, or perhaps only malaise. But if we ignore these comparatively mild warnings, the danger will inevitably become more and more acute and then—though perhaps in a less dramatic form—we shall sooner or later be confronted with a situation nearly akin to the one depicted in this book.

Extrasensory perception—one could use a whole seminar on this aspect alone of the horse. We already touched on it in the *Iliad* where

Xanthus foretells Achilles' death, and we must just mention Sleipnir, Wotan's eight-legged horse (see *Symbole der Wandlung* for illustration).[11] Jung says, in connection with Wotan and Sleipnir—he even calls Wotan half-human, half-horse, so closely is he united with Sleipnir:

> Legends attribute qualities to horses that belong psychologically to the unconscious of man. Horses are clairvoyant and (supernaturally) sharp of hearing, they show us the way when we are lost and cannot help ourselves, they have mantic (divinatory) power; in the *Iliad* it is the horse that foresees the fatal event; they hear the words spoken by the corpse being carried to the grave which man cannot hear. Caesar hears from his human-footed horse that he will conquer the world.[12]

The ESP aspect is the direct opposite of panic, for it is well known that such communications can only be heard if we are very quiet for they tend to be "a still small voice" that is only too easy to drown.

Dr. von Franz drew my attention to one of the best horse fairy stories that I ever read. It is called "The Magic Horse" and is to be found in the Turkestan volume of fairy stories.[13] Unfortunately, there is only time to take the last image, which makes an excellent conclusion to our theme, and to give you the barest outline of the story.

In the story, there is a king with a beautiful daughter whom he does not want to lose, so he feeds up a flea until it becomes as big as an elephant, after which he skins it. He then sets suitors for the hand of the princess the riddle that they shall guess what the skin is. No one can guess, but a djinn who lives in a lake hears a servant say that it was a pity that no one knows that it is the skin of a flea. The king does not want to give his daughter to the djinn, who has now been able to give the answer, but the latter has magic power and makes such terrible weather that he has to give in. The princess makes difficulties, but he has to submit and also has to choose a dowry. When she goes into the stable, a little magic horse says, "Choose me," then he names four magic objects which they should take with them, namely a mirror, a comb, salt, and a carnation. It is the djinn's intention to run off with the girl and eat her, but the little horse makes her throw away the magic objects, each of which makes a different obstacle which the djinn has to get by, and so each time they gain a little more time. The last object, the mirror,

---

[11]*CW* 5, par. 421.

[12]Ibid.

[13]"Das Zauberros," *Marchen aus Turkestan und Tibet*, Diedrich, Jena, 1933, p. 126ff.

makes a river, and the princess tells the djinn that the only way to cross is by putting stones around one's neck, and so the djinn sinks to the bottom of the river and is drowned. The princess and the little horse then arrive in another country, and the king there falls in love with her for her beauty and marries her. They are happy until the king goes hunting when the (resurrected) djinn manages to get hold of a letter which is being sent the king to say that the queen has beautiful twin boys. The djinn changes the sense of the letter and says that she has given birth to a cat and a dog, but the king replies that they are all to be taken care of until he arrives. This letter the djinn also changes into one which says that she is to be driven out with her children into the wilderness. This is done. The djinn goes with her, and when they are by a river, he says he is now going to eat her children. She knows that if she throws the hairs of the horse into a fire, the horse will appear, and she therefore persuades the djinn to light a fire to cook the children. He does so, she throws in the hairs, the horse appears and fights with the djinn and eventually overcomes him. The horse then makes the princess kill him and put his head on one side, his legs in the four directions of the compass, and throw away his entrails. She is then to sit with her children under the ribs. When she has done this the legs turn into beautiful golden poplars with emerald leaves, the entrails become villages and fields, etc., the ribs a beautiful golden castle, and the head a silvery stream of pure water. After a long time, the king finds her and they live together in this mandala which originally was the horse.

Here the extrasensory perception, in a particularly subtle and positive form, is used to free the girl from the danger of possession by the negative animus and, in addition, the horse reveals the *goal* of ESP in general, i.e., the mandala, the totality, the Self. Already an indication of this is to be found in the square of Pegasus but here it goes much further: the horse itself becomes a particularly differentiated form of mandala.

What in the beginning seems to be physical, namely the horse instinct at the infrared end of the scale, reveals here the ultraviolet aspect far more completely than we have seen it before, the meaning of the archetypal image, the process of individuation itself. From this image, we can even postulate that if we live the natural flow of our life completely, including the sacrifice, we arrive naturally at the goal which is hidden in the horse.

It is particularly interesting that it is the horse itself which insists on the sacrifice here and which suggests that the *libido itself contains its own spiritual counterpart*, that it sublimates itself, so to speak (in contradistinction to the Freudian idea of our having to sublimate our instincts). The horse here sacrifices itself if we have the courage to accept the intense suffering involved in the sacrifice as the princess eventually does in this story.

We see very closely here the feminine quality of the horse, for though it is the guide, on account of its unusual ESP, it carries us and even contains us, as is clear in this story and in the Brihadaranyaka Upanishad. The horse, in contrast to the cat or dog, here reveals itself as not only libido and its goal, but also as the vessel in which the whole process takes place.

CONCLUSION

We have raced through a fragment of the rich symbolism with which the archetypal images of our three animals have confronted us and seen something, at all events, of their many-sided meaning.

I should like to conclude with a few words on the qualities of the instincts which all these animals have in common and those which are specific to each. All three are represented by domesticated animals, therefore we have been dealing with instincts that are near to us, with all of which we can establish a connection. (I need not remind you of the many animals, birds, insects, reptiles, and so on that represent the more distant or deeper layers of instincts that are also connected with our psyche.)

Animals in general seem to represent the lower instinctive forces in man which often know the way when our conscious is entirely at sea. This has turned out to be true of all our three animals; of all of them we can say that "if we follow the way of nature, it will lead us to our own law," or we can apply Christ's logion to them all and say that they are among those that "lead us to the kingdom of heaven." In other words, we could say that all instincts serve the process of individuation in some form or other, that this goal is common to them all, and that their negative aspects are only constellated when we are not serving this goal ourselves. For instance, the cat instinct only degenerates into cattiness when we are being untrue to the process of individuation and so on, with other aspects and animals.

Something also which is common to all is the fact that we cannot project human notions of right and wrong onto any of them, yet it is just the animal that confronts us with the greatest moral problem, for everything depends on our right or wrong attitude to it. Here it is useful to remember Lorenz's dream of the baby rats and to search for a deep instinctive feeling of what we can or cannot do in order to understand any of our three. They all belong to the human nature, to the luminosities that surround our ego, and all three can help us when our consciousness is entirely at fault.

Of all our three animals, the horse comes the nearest to being the representative of what the instincts in general can do for us. The horse is a far wider and more embracing symbol than cat or dog, but, on the other hand, the two last are much more specific and have a narrower and more definite meaning.

I know of no example in fairy stories or mythology where the cat or the dog becomes the mandala, where they represent the vessel in which the whole process takes place. (There may be exceptions but I do not know one, nor does Dr. von Franz. They are relatively rare at all events.) The cat and the dog represent helpful instincts that guide us within the mandala or help us to find our way back when we have strayed outside.

The cat is the least related of our three animals, it walks by itself and must be allowed to do so in order that this instinct can work in us in its most positive form. We shall never really domesticate this instinct but must rather regard it as something which remains wild in us, which can yet work for the good of the whole if we can find the *right attitude to it.*

On the other hand, the cat is the smallest and most harmless of the three, it can do us very little harm in comparison with a fierce dog or unruly horse and this, of course, also has a bearing on the right attitude toward it. As we saw, cats are often treated with the utmost cruelty, and naturally, if we fall into this error, we have no chance whatever of enlisting the assistance of the cat instinct.

The dog is the most related of all our animals and, as against the cat and the horse, very rarely reverts willingly to the wild state. We are for the most part the home center to which its elastic band is attached, and this makes an enormous difference to our connection with the dog instinct. The enormous quantity of myths and fairy stories where dogs become human (the motif is found with other animals but is commonest with the dog) show us how near this instinct is to us and how much of it we can assimilate. But above all, it is a matter of *relating* to the dog, and if we can achieve this, he will be our guide to the beyond and in the unconscious, and we shall be able to deal with him as the watchdog of heaven (as on the Cinvat Bridge) or as Cerberus guarding the door of hell. He also has the greatest healing power of any of the three, as seen in the role which he played in the cult of Aesculapius.

Our attitude to the horse, and our horse instinct, is somewhere in between that which is advisable to cat and dog. The horse is not so completely independent as the cat, nor so dependent on our relationship as the dog. In contrast to the two others, it is much stronger than we are, it can carry and even contain us, as we have seen. We must domesticate, learn to ride and drive it, and yet we must let it follow its own law, for Pegasus has the square, the totality, and the horse is the symbol *par excellence* for the libido that is leading us—through sacrifice—to the mandala, to the Self.

As I hope has been clear throughout, the whole functional meaning of all three animals depends on our attitude to them; as domestic animals they are all three factors for which we carry the responsibility. If we meet a starving lion in a dream, for instance, we are not responsible for the fact that it has had no food, but if we meet any of our animals in the same condition, we can be sure that we are responsible and that the dream is drawing our attention to some neglect on the part of consciousness. It is just the instincts, therefore, as represented by domestic animals that are especially important, and the myths which deal with them make an appeal, as it were, to our understanding and sense of responsibility towards these animals.

In our time, when the problem of the instincts has become so red hot, it is necessary to start at the end where we are able to do something about it, so that the right interpretation of our animals—when they appear in dreams or active imagination—is particularly important.

BIBLIOGRAPHY

IN TUNE WITH THE UNCONSCIOUS: A PORTRAIT OF BARBARA HANNAH

Hannah, Barbara. *Encounters with the Soul: Active Imagination.* Santa Monica, Calif.: Sigo Press, 1981.

______. *Jung, His Life and Work: A Biographical Memoir.* New York: G. P. Putnam's Sons, 1976.

______. *Striving Toward Wholeness.* New York: G. P. Putnam's Sons, 1971.

______. "The Beyond," Bailey Island Lecture, Maine, 1962.

Hoffman, Barbara. "Review of *Jung, His Life and Work: A Biographical Memoir*, by Barbara Hannah." *Best Sellers* (March 1977).

"Review of Barbara Hannah's Lecture," *Bulletin of the Analytical Psychology Club of New York,* 1952.

THE BEYOND

Jung, C. G. *Memories, Dreams, Reflections.* New York: Pantheon Books, 1961.

______. "The Visions of Zosimos." In *The Collected Works of C. G. Jung,* vol. 13. Princeton, N.J.: Princeton University Press, 1967.

______. "Concerning Rebirth." In *CW*, vol. 9i. Princeton, N.J.: Princeton University Press, 1959.

Hauer, J. W. "Kundalini Yoga." Seminar at Psychological Club, Zurich, 1932.

Wilhelm, Richard. *The Secret of the Golden Flower.* London: Routledge and Kegan Paul, 1931, reprinted 1965, 1967, 1969.

______. "Death and Renewal in China." *Spring* (1962): 20–44.

Evans, P. deB., trans. *Meister Eckhart.* London: John Watkins, reprinted 1952.

CAT, DOG, AND HORSE SEMINAR

Bonnet, H. *Reallexikon der Aegyptischen Religionsgeschichte.* Berlin: Walter de Gruyter and Co., 1952.

Budge, E. A. *The Book of the Dead,* 2nd ed. rev. New York: E. P. Dutton and Co., 1928.

Brehm, A. E. *Thierleben.* Leipzig: Verlag des Bibliographischen Instituts, 1876–1878.

Christie, Agatha. *Come Tell Me Where You Live.* New York: Dodd, 1946.

Cunningham, Graham. *Rodeo.* Garden City, N.Y.: Doubleday, Doran and Co., 1936.

Erman, Adolf. *Die Religion der Aegypter.* Berlin: Walter de Gruyter and Co., 1934.

Gaidoz, "A propos des chiens d'Epidaure." In *Revue Archeologique,* 1884.

Gubernatis, A. de. *Zoological Mythology or the Legends of Animals,* 2 vols. London: Trubner and Co., 1872.

Hogg, James. *Private Memoirs and Confessions of a Justified Sinner.* New York: W. W. Norton and Co., 1970.

Homer, *The Iliad,* A. T. Murray, trans. Cambridge, Mass.: Harvard University Press, 1925.

Howey, M. Oldfield. *The Horse in Magic and Myth.* London: W. Rider and Son, 1923.

Jung, C. G. *Answer to Job. CW,* vol. 11. Princeton, N.J.: Princeton University Press, 1958.

_____. "Instinct and the Unconscious." In *CW,* vol. 8. Princeton, N.J.: Princeton University Press, 1957.

_____. "On the Nature of the Psyche." In *CW,* vol. 8. Princeton, N.J.: Princeton University Press, 1957.

_____. *Psychological Analysis of Neitzsche's Zarathustra.* Zurich: Spring, 1934–1939.

_____. *Psychology and Alchemy. CW,* vol. 12. Princeton, N.J.: Princeton University Press, 1953.

_____. *Symbols of Transformation. CW,* vol. 5. Princeton, N.J.: Princeton University Press, 1956.

_____. "Synchronicity: An Acausal Connecting Principle." In *CW,* vol. 8. Princeton, N.J.: Princeton University Press, 1957.

_____. "The Phenomenology of the Spirit in Fairytales." In *CW,* vol. 9i. Princeton, N.J.: Princeton University Press, 1959.

———. *The Visions Seminars*. Zurich: Spring Publications, 1976.

———. "Transformation Symbolism in the Mass." In *CW*, vol. 11. Princeton, N.J.: Princeton University Press, 1958.

Jung, C. G., and C. Kerenyi. *Essays on a Science of Mythology*. Princeton, N.J.: Princeton University Press, 1949.

Jungbauer, G., ed. *Marchen aus Turkestan und Tibet*. "Das Zauberros," no. 9. Jena: Eugen Diederich Verlag, 1923.

Kretschmar, F. *Hundesstammvater und Kerberos*, 2 vols. Stuttgart: Strecker und Schroder, 1938.

Lorenz, K. *So kam der Mensch auf den Hund*. Vienna: Verlag Dr. G. Borotha, 1950.

Märchen aus Turkestan und Tibet. "Das Zauberros," (Jena: Eugen Diederichs Verlag, 1923.

Plato. *Five Dialogues*. 3rd ed. A. D. Lindsay, trans. New York: E. P. Dutton and Co., 1917.

Reinach, "Las Chiens dans le Culte d'Esculape." In *Revue Archeologique*, 1884.

Scharf-Kluger, R. *Satan in the Old Testament*. H. Nagel, trans. Evanston, Ill.: Northwestern University Press, 1967.

von Franz, M.-L. *"Archetypal Patterns in Fairy Tales."* Lectures. Zurich: C. G. Jung Institute, 1951.

Wilhelm, R. "Death and Renewal." J. A. Pratt, trans. *Spring* (1962): 20–44.

Williams, J. H. *Elephant Bill*. London, 1952.

Lectures and Manuscripts of Barbara Hannah

AT THE C. G. JUNG INSTITUTE, ZÜRICH

"Active Imagination," record of a talk given in Zürich, September 25, 1967.
"All's Well That Ends Well," *Spring* (1956).
"Animus Figures in Literature and Modern Life," lecture at the C. G. Jung Institute, Zurich, 1953.
"The Beyond," lecture at the Second Bailey Island Conference, in honor of Esther Harding's 80th Birthday, August, 1968.
"Cat, Dog, and Horse Seminar," April 26, 1954.
"Ego and Shadow," lecture 85, Guild of Pastoral Psychology, London, March, 1955.
"Possession and Exorcism: Polarities of the Psyche," five lectures, 1956.
"Problem of Contact with the Animus," lecture 70, Guild of Pastoral Psychology, London, February 16, 1951.
"The Problem of Women's Plots in 'The Evil Vineyard,'" lecture 51, Guild of Pastoral Psychology, London, June 15, 29, 1946.
"Religious Function of the Animus in the Book of Tobit," lecture 114, Guild of Pastoral Psychology, London, October 7, 1960.
"Some Remarks on Active Imagination," *Spring* (1953).
"Victims of the Creative Spirit: A Contribution to the Psychology of the Brontës from the Jungian Point of View," lecture 68, Guild of Pastoral Psychology, London, July 21, 1950.
"Women's Plots," lecture at the C. G. Jung Institute, Zürich, November, 1970.

AT THE PSYCHOLOGICAL CLUB, ZÜRICH

"Referat Uber Esther Harding's Frauenmysterium"
"The Brontës and Modern Women"
"The Evil Vineyard"
"St. Victor's Conversation with the Anima"
"A Case of Possession and Exorcism"

PUBLISHED BOOKS

Jung, His Life and Work: A Biographical Memoir. New York: G. P. Putnam's Sons, 1976.

Encounters with the Soul: Active Imagination as Developed by C. G. Jung. Santa Monica, Calif.: Sigo Press, 1981.

Striving Toward Wholeness. New York: G. P. Putnam's Sons, 1971.

INDEX

Made in the USA
Monee, IL
08 November 2026

67384894R00090